普通高等教育"十一五"国家级规划教材
全国高等医药院校药学类实验双语教材

中药制剂学实验与指导

（供药学类、中药学类专业用）

主编 赵浩如

编者 （按姓氏笔画排名）

王宇薪 石心红 刘利根
刘晓华 汤明辉 林以宁
黄罗生 富志军

协编 杨永刚 钱韵旭 邓丹丹
卓 佳 殷晓东 梁待亮

中国医药科技出版社

感谢外籍英文教授 Ellen Riorden 对本书的英文提出的宝贵意见。

全国高等医药院校药学类规划教材常务编委会

出版说明

全国高等医药院校药学类专业规划教材是目前国内体系最完整、专业覆盖最全面、作者队伍最权威的药学类教材。随着我国药学教育事业的快速发展，药学及相关专业办学规模和水平的不断扩大和提高，课程设置的不断更新，对药学类教材的质量提出了更高的要求。

全国高等医药院校药学类规划教材编写委员会在调查和总结上轮药学类规划教材质量和使用情况的基础上，经过审议和规划，组织中国药科大学、沈阳药科大学、广东药学院、北京大学药学院、复旦大学药学院、四川大学华西药学院、北京中医药大学、西安交通大学医学院、华中科技大学同济药学院、山东大学药学院、山西医科大学药学院、第二军医大学药学院、山东中医药大学、上海中医药大学和江西中医学院等数十所院校的教师共同进行药学类第三轮规划教材的编写修订工作。

药学类第三轮规划教材的编写修订，坚持紧扣药学类专业本科教育培养目标，参考执业药师资格准入标准，强调药学特色鲜明，体现现代医药科技水平，进一步提高教材水平和质量。同时，针对学生自学、复习、考试等需要，紧扣主干教材内容，新编了相应的学习指导与习题集等配套教材。

本套教材由中国医药科技出版社出版，供全国高等医药院校药学类及相关专业使用。其中包括理论课教材82种，实验课教材38种，配套教材10种，其中有45种入选普通高等教育“十一五”国家级规划教材。

全国高等医药院校药学类规划教材

编写委员会

2009年8月1日

序

实验教学是高等药学院校最基本的教学形式之一，对培养学生科学的思维与方法、创新意识与能力，全面推进素质教育有着重要的作用。飞速发展的科学技术，已成为主导社会进步的重要因素。高等药学院校必须不断更新教学内容，以学科发展的前沿知识充实实验课程内容。

近年来，中国药科大学坚持以研究促教改，通过承担教育部“世行贷款——21世纪初高等教育教学改革项目”及立项校内教改课题等多种方式，调动了广大教师投身教学改革的积极性，将转变教师的教育思想观念与教学内容、教学方法的改革紧密结合起来，取得了实效。此次推出的国家“十五”规划教材——药学专业双语实验教学系列，是广大教师长期钻研实验课程教学体系，改革教学内容，实现教育创新的重要成果。他们站在21世纪教育、科技和社会发展趋势的高度，对药学专业实验课程的教学内容进行了“精选”、“整合”和“创新”，强调对学生的动手能力、创新思维、科学素养等综合素质的全面培养。这套教材具有以下的特点：

1．教材将各学科的实验内容进行了广泛的“精选”，既体现了高等药学教育“面向世界、面向未来、面向现代化”，也考虑到我国药学教育的现状与实际；既体现了各门实验课程自身的独立性、系统性和科学性，又充分考虑到各门实验课程之间的联系与衔接，有助于学生在教学大纲规定的实验教学学时内掌握基本操作技术，提高动手能力，养成严谨、求实、创新的科学态度。

2．教材中新增的综合性、设计性实验有利于学生全面了解和综合掌握本门实验课程的教学内容。这一举措既满足了学生个性发展的需要，更注重培养学生分析问题、解决问题的能力和创新意识。

3．教材中适当安排一些反映药学学科发展前沿的实验，有利于学生在掌握实验基本技术的同时，对药学学科的新进展、新技术有所了解，激发他们学习药学知识与相关学科的兴趣。

4．教材以实践教学为突破口，采用双语体系编写，为实验课程改革构建数字化、信息化和外语教学的平台，有利于提高学生的科技英语水平。通过我校多年的药学系列实验课程双语教学实践，证明学生完全能够接受此套教材的教学。

国家十五规划教材——药学专业双语实验教学系列教材的陆续出版，必将对推动我国高等药学教育的健康发展，产生积极而深远的影响。由于采用双语体系编写药学教学实验丛书尚属首次，缺乏经验，在内容选择及编写方法上的不妥之处，在所难免。欢迎从事药学教育的同行们批评赐教。

吴晓明

（中国药科大学校长、博士、教授、博士生导师）

2003 年 1 月于南京

Preface

Experimental teaching is one of the most fundamental teaching means in pharmaceutical colleges, playing an important role in training scientific thoughts and methods, creative consciousness and ability of the students as well as in promoting quality - oriented education in all - round way. Fast - advancing science and technology has come to be an important factor in dominating social progress. Teaching materials must be updated continually in pharmaceutical colleges, especially enriching the materials of experimental courses with the most advanced knowledge in the subject.

In recent years, China Pharmaceutical University have been stressing the promotion of teaching reform on the basis of research, succeeding in stimulating teachers' enthusiasm for teaching reform by various means such as undertaking the project of teaching reform in higher education at the beginning of 21st century sponsored financially by World Bank and entrusted by the Ministry of Education as well as approving and ratifying internal programs on teaching reform. Meanwhile, it yields fruits to integrate the transforming of teachers' educational ideology into the reform of teaching materials and methods. This series of textbook of national "Tenth - five" planning - bilingual pharmaceutical experimental teaching series, is an important achievement made through studying ueaching system of experimental courses for long, reforming teaching materials and carrying out educational innovation of all the teachers concerned.

Meeting the new demands for education, science and technology and social growth, they select, integrate and innovate the teaching materials of pharmaceutical experimental courses, stressing the overall cultivation of comprehensive qualities, including experimental ability, creative thought and scientific attainments. This set of textbook possesses the following features:

1. These textbooks make an extensive "selection" of the experimental materials of each subject, reflecting the goal of facing the world, facing the future and facing the modernization in higher pharmaceutical education, and taking into account the status quota and reality of our pharmaceutical education; meanwhile embodying the individuality, systematicness and scientificalness of each experimental courses, which helps the students to grasp basic techniques of operation within the class hours of experimental teaching prescribed by teaching syllabus and to improve their experimental ability and finally to cultivate a scientific approach of precision, practicality and creation.

2. The comprehensive designing experiments newly supplemented in the textbooks help the students to learn totally and grasp comprehensively the teaching materials of the experimental courses, which not only meets the students' needs for individual development but also trains their ability to analyze and solve problems and cultivates their creative consciousness.

3. Some experiments representing the latest development in pharmacy are properly included in the textbooks, which helps the students to learn about new advance and technology in pharmacy and to further arouse their interests in studying pharmacy and relevant subjects while grasping some basic techniques of experiment.

4. The textbooks take experimental teaching as starting point and are compiled in a system of bilingualism and aim to set up a platform of digitalization, information and foreign language teaching for the purpose of reforming experimental courses, which serves to enhance the students' level of technological English. It has been proved that the students have no difficulty being adapted to the teaching of this set of textbook through many years of bilingual teaching practice carried out in a series of pharmaceutical experimental courses of our university.

The successive publishing of the series of textbooks used for bilingual pharmaceutical experimental teaching – the national "Tenth—five" planning textbooks, will surely produce good and far – reaching influence in promoting the sound development of higher pharmaceutical education of our country. Since it is the first time that we have compiled this series of textbook of pharmaceutical teaching experiment in a bilingual system, we lack experience and thus some defects in choice of materials and way of compilation are inevitable. Experts engaged in pharmaceutical education are welcome to give any criticisms and advice.

Wu Xiaoming

Ph. D, prof., and supervisor of doctoral candidates
President of China Pharmaceutical University
Nanjing
Jan, 2003

目　　录

第一章　绪　论

一、前言

本实验讲义中所写的每个实验是一类中药制剂（固体、液体、半固体或分散体系）的一般代表性制剂或者制剂技术。由于制剂学涉及的剂型品种和制剂技术以及制剂设备很多，我们不可能在有限的学时中涵盖所有的内容。选择这些实验是为了说明和加强在课堂讲授的中药药剂学规定的概念，向学生介绍各类制剂的化学、制备、质量控制和应用的基本要素。在该讲义中所练习的制剂实验选自正式的收载药品标准和规范的典籍：2000 年版《中华人民共和国药典》（简称《中国药典》）1997 年英文版《中国药典》和国家食品药品监督管理局（卫生部）药品标准，以期能有助于学生掌握国家标准对各种中药制剂的一般要求。

本书每章的要求不相同，其格式也不一定相同。为了达到教学目的，尽可能学好这些实验课，避免不了解情况产生的尴尬，要求每个学生在课前熟悉将要进行的实验，认真阅读课文及其注释的参考文献，并且回答有关问题。学生在学习的时候发挥主观能动性是必要的。

为了减少本书的成本，我们省略了本书用到的有关仪器设备和辅料的图示和说明。这些仪器设备和辅料可以在教科书《中药药剂学》和《中国药典》中找到，并且其中有详细的说明。

本书有关药物的内容仅供学生作为实验练习用，如有其他用途请读者阅读有关正式标准。

该实验讲义中的实验随着中药制剂学的发展可以进行适当地修改。我们用两种语言为学生出版了该讲义。教师可以根据他们为学生设置的课程的需要从该讲义中选择实验内容。我们欢迎读者对本书中有关技术和语言问题提出宝贵意见。

二、教学目标

在完成既定的课程学习任务后，学生应该在下列方面达到一定的水平：

1. 通过对仪器设备的实际操作，能够学会一定的中药生产工艺的技能。
2. 能够说明《中华人民共和国药典》对各类中药制剂的要求。
3. 懂得曾学习过的中成药的医疗用途。
4. 能够解释曾学习过的中药配方中的成分的作用和剂量。
5. 懂得所学习的药物是否能用其他剂型给药。

6．懂得制剂中可能影响疗效的活性成分的性质（例如，黄芩苷是小儿消炎栓中的黄芩的活性成分，具有易于被氧化的性质。应该知道在生产和储藏该制剂时，如何防止黄芩苷被氧化）。

三、学生实验须知

1．个人应保持整洁，在实验室期间应穿干净的实验室工作服。

2．学生应在自已的实验台工作并保持安静，不得无故离开。

3．不得将食物或饮料带入实验室，以保证安全。

4．每位学生在实验前应研究预期要上的实验课内容。通过课前阅读课文、参考资料、填写必要的实验报告内容（例如，题目、要求等）和回答问题，熟悉实验课要学习的内容。

5．天平、玻璃仪器和其他设备需要实验经费购买，来之不易。学习正确地使用这些仪器设备，并且注意爱护它们。

6．请勿将不溶性固体、油脂或者软膏倒入洗涤池。可以将这些东西用纸包裹后放入垃圾桶内。

7．请勿浪费或过量使用药物或化学试剂。按照规定的方法操作。不正确的操作，可能带来危险。除非得到老师的许可，请勿将取出的过量的材料返回原来储藏的容器中，以免污染。

8．每位同学都有责任保持实验室的整洁。在使用并且清洁完毕后，将玻璃仪器和其他设备妥善地复归原处，以备其他同学使用。

9．学生应该在规定的时间内完成实验。如果确实因为生病或其他原因不能上课，必须在实验前向指导老师请假（意外事故除外）。

10．完成的产品必须经指导老师检查或评分后，然后倒掉或放在合适的容器中。

11．不得将实验室产品、药物和试剂带走使用，以维护公共财产和人身安全。

12．在实验室发生任何意外事件，请立即报告指导老师。

13．应公示学生的卫生值班名单。

14．如果本须知与学校的规定相冲突，则学生应服从学校的规定。

四、实验报告和成绩

每个实验结束后，学生都应写一份书面报告，其内容包括一个制剂工作的内容摘要和实验资料（如下所示）。该报告也可包含你认为重要的信息。在报告内容的前面应有一页封面，请写上实验题目、你的姓名、学号、班级和实验日期。

报告中的实验资料

1．处方和分析	所有制剂成分的名称、数量和作用
2．实验方法	每一个步骤的详细说明，包括必要的计算
3．包装和贮藏	容器类型、温度、光线等内容

续表

4. 标识资料	成品标签上应有的说明
5. 物理化学资料	与制备和质量控制有关的药物活性成分的说明
6. 检查资料	对你所制备的成品的检查方法和结果

对于那些有产品的实验，学生应准备所有产品的标签并且正确地贴好。对每位学生的实验都将给出成绩。成绩的判定基于所制备的制剂质量、实验报告、相应的技术以及实验室表现。每堂实验课开始时可能有一个测验。该测验包括目前的和以前的实验课内容，以及任何有关实验产品和方法的问题。

五、参考书

1. 张兆旺，中药药剂学．北京：中国中医药出版社，2003
2. 屠锡德等，药剂学（第三版）．北京：人民卫生出版社，2002
3. 国家药典委员会，中华人民共和国药典

Pharmaceutics of Traditional Chinese Medicine (TCM) Laboratory Course

Introduction

Each laboratory exercise collected in this manual is generally representative of a class of TCM preparations (solid, liquid, semisolid, or disperse systems), or a pharmaceutical technique. Pharmaceutics ranges over a large numbers of dosage forms, technological processes, and equipment. The proposed exercises cannot over much of the content with a limited course. The exercises have been chosen either to illustrate and reinforce a specific concept discussed in the lecture portion of the *Pharmaceutics of Traditional Chinese Medicine (TCM)* course and to introduce the student to the pharmaceutical uses, design, methods of preparation, ingredients, and evaluation of the various classes of dosage forms. Preparations in this manual are mostly chose from official compendia which provide the standards and specifications for various pharmaceutical preparations, including the *Pharmacopoeia of the People's Republic of China* (2000) (abbreviated as the Chinese Pharmacopoeia; Ch.P.), the *Pharmacopoeia of the People's Republic of China* (English edition, 1997), and the SFDA (Ministry of Health) Drug Standards, which are designed and expected to help understand the general requirements of each TCM dosage forms complied with the national standards.

The requirement of each chapter for students is different as well as its format. To achieve the objective of study, optimize the learning experience, and avoid the natural frustration in unknown situations, each student is required to become familiar with the laboratory exercise that will be conducted by reading it over, reading the references cited in the text, and answering the respective questions before the laboratory period.

To minimize the cost of this book, we deleted all the illustrations of equipment and excipients used in this manual. They can be found in the book *Pharmaceutics of Traditional Chinese Medicine* for the lecture course and in the *Chinese Pharmacopoeia* with more detail.

The description and statement about any drugs recorded in this book applies only the students' laboratory exercises. For more information the reader should read the related official standards.

Laboratory exercises in this manual may be revised properly according the development in the field. We publish the material in a bilingual edition for students. Teachers may select laboratory exercises from this manual to construct their own course for students. However we would appreciate any suggestions from our readers on issues both of the technology and language in the book. Thank you.

Course Goals

Upon completion of the learning activities in this course, the student should be able to perform the following objectives at the specified level:

1. Develop skills and techniques that are part of TCM pharmaceutical procedures through the actual use of equipment and instruments.

2. Interpret requirements for a TCM preparation in the *Pharmacopeia of the People's Republic of China*.

3. Know the therapeutic use of the finished product you have worked on.

4. Explain the actions and doses of each botanical ingredient in a TCM formulation you have learned.

5. Know if the drug under study can be administered in some other dosage form.

6. Identify the properties of the active ingredient in the dosage form that may influence the therapeutic effect. (e.g. Baicalin, an active constituent of radix scutellariae in Xiao' er Xiaoyan suppository, has a property with which it is liable to become oxidized. Know how to protect the preparation in manufacture and storage from oxidization.)

Laboratory Notice to Students

1. Personal cleanliness and neatness are always necessary. Each student must wear a clean laboratory coat at all times while in the laboratory.

2. Each student is to work quietly at his own desk unless he/she has a good reason to be somewhere else.

3. No food items or drinks can be brought into the lab.

4. Study each experiment before attempting to do the work. Each student is required to become familiar with each laboratory exercise by reading it over, reading the reference information, filling out the necessary part of the preparation report (e. g., title, objectives), and answering the respective questions BEFORE the laboratory period.

5. Balances, glassware and other equipment are bought with the experiment fund and has not come easily. Learn to use them correctly and take care of them.

6. Do not place insoluble solids, oils or ointments in the sink. Wrap these in paper towels and place in a waste container.

7. Please do not waste or use excessive amounts of drugs or chemicals. Use them according to the specified methods. Incorrect operation of an experiment may be dangerous. Never return any excess material from a stock container unless advised to do so by the instructor. There is danger of contamination.

8. Each student is responsible for the neat and clean appearance of the lab. Return all

glassware, apparatus and equipment to their proper locations after they are properly cleaned and are ready for use by other students.

9. Work in a laboratory section within the permitted time. If you must miss a lab because of illness or another reason, notify the course instructor before the lab, exceptions made for accidents.

10. Completed products should be checked or graded by the instructor and the contents should be poured out or placed in the proper receptacle.

11. Do not remove any produce, drugs or chemicals from the laboratory for personal use. This is to ensure safety for public property and persons.

12. All accidents in the laboratory most be immediately reported to the instructor.

13. A roster will be posted for cleaning assignments.

14. The students should comply with the regulation of the university. If this manual in any way conflicts with them, please ask your instructor.

Experiment Reports and Grades

For each laboratory exercise, the student will prepare a written report including an abstract of the dosage form being prepared and the following Experimental Information. You may include any additional information in your report that you consider to be important. Please include a cover sheet having your name, lab day, student identification number, class identification number and laboratory title.

Experimental Information in the Report

1. Formula	Complete listing of all ingredients, amounts and uses.
2. Method of Preparation	Step – by – step detailed instructions, with calculations
3. Packaging and Storage	Container type, temperature, light, etc. considerations
4. Labeling Information	Special instructions for the label of the finished product.
5. Physicochemical Information	Description of active constituents of the herbs, relating to manufacture and control.
6. Test Information	Test methods and results of the finished product you prepared

For laboratory exercises that contain products, each of you will prepare and properly label all of the products. Each individual student will receive a grade for your laboratory exercises. The grade will be based on the quality of the preparation prepared, the experiment report, proper technique and on laboratory practice.

Each laboratory session may begin with a quiz. The quiz will cover the previous and the present laboratory session, and any questions on products and procedures.

Reference Books

1. Zhang Zhaowang, Pharmaceutics of Traditional Chinese Medicine. Beijing: China

Press of Traditional Chinese Medicine，2003

2. Tu Xide，et al.，Pharmaceutics (3rd edition). Beijing: People's Press of Health，2002

3. Pharmacopoeia Committee of PRC，Pharmacopoeia of the People's Republic of China

实验一　酊　　剂

【实验目的】

掌握渗漉法操作及酊剂的制备。

【实验指导】

酊剂[1]是指药物用规定浓度的乙醇提取或溶解而制成的澄清液体制剂，亦可用流浸膏稀释制成。

1．酊剂在生产与贮藏期间应符合下列有关规定

（1）除另有规定外，含有毒性药或强效药的酊剂，每100ml应相当于原药材10g；其他酊剂，一般每100ml相当于原药材20g。

（2）含有毒性药的酊剂，其有效成分明确者，可以根据其半成品的含量加以调整。

（3）酊剂可用溶解法、稀释法、浸渍法或渗漉法制备。

溶解法或稀释法　取药物粉末或流浸膏，加规定浓度的乙醇适量，溶解或稀释，静置，必要时滤过，即得。

浸渍法　取适当粉碎的药材，置有盖容器中，加入溶剂适量，密盖，搅拌或振摇，浸渍3～5日或规定的时间，倾取上清液，再加入溶剂适量，依法浸渍至有效成分充分浸出，合并浸出液，加溶剂至规定量后，静置24小时，滤过，即得。

渗漉法　根据药材的性质选用圆柱形或圆锥形的渗漉器。取适当粉碎的药材加溶剂均匀湿润，密闭放置一定时间，再装入渗漉器渗漉。收集85%药材量的初漉液另器保存，渗漉液经低温浓缩后与初漉液合并，调整至规定量，静置24小时，滤过，即得。

（4）酊剂久置产生沉淀时，在乙醇和有效成分含量符合各该品种规定的情况下，可滤过除去沉淀。

（5）酊剂应置遮光容器内密闭，在阴凉处贮藏。

2．酊剂的检查

乙醇量检查　参见《中华人民共和国药典》附录。

甲醇量检查　每1L供试液含甲醇量不得超过0.4g。检查方法参见《中华人民共和国药典》附录。

实验　姜　　酊

姜酊是中华人民共和国药典收载的中药制剂[2]。姜酊由干姜浸膏制成。干姜来源于姜 *Zingiber officinale* Rosc. 的干燥根茎，含挥发油2%～3.5%。

性状：本品为淡黄色的液体；有姜的香气，味辣。

功能与主治：健胃驱风药。

用法与用量：口服，一次2～4ml，一日6～12ml。

贮藏：密封。

【实验材料】

仪器：烧杯、滤纸、圆锥形渗漉器、漏斗。

药品和试剂：姜粉（10~20目）、90%乙醇等。

【实验方法】

1．处方

姜粉	200g
90%乙醇	适量
共制成	1000ml

2．制备

（1）姜流浸膏的制备

浸泡　取干燥姜粉（10~20目）20g，用15ml 90%乙醇拌匀湿润后密闭放置24小时。取脱脂棉一团，用浸出液湿润后垫在渗漉器底部，将浸渍的姜粉分次装入渗漉器内，每次装入适量后均压紧压平。装完后用滤纸或纱布覆盖药材面，并加入一些重物（如玻璃珠、石块）。

渗漉　打开渗漉筒浸液出口活塞，向渗漉筒内缓缓加入90%乙醇，待溶液自出口流出时，关闭活塞，流出的溶媒再倒入筒内，加溶媒使溶媒面高出药粉数厘米，加盖放置24小时。以每1000克每分钟2~4ml流出液的速度渗漉，渗漉过程中需随时补充溶媒，使药材中有效成分充分浸出。收集初漉液17ml，放入有盖容器中。继续渗漉至渗漉液接近无色、姜的香气和辣味已淡薄为止，收集续漉液。

浓缩过滤　在60℃以下浓缩至稠膏状，加入初漉液，混合，滤过。

（2）姜酊的配制

稀释配液　取姜流浸膏20ml，用90%乙醇稀释至100ml，静置24小时，俟澄清，过滤，即得。

3．含量测定

姜流浸膏的醚溶性物质不得少于4.5%（参见《中国药典》之姜流浸膏）。

4．检查

乙醇量　按照《中国药典》附录之乙醇量测定法的蒸馏法第一法测定。姜酊的乙醇量应为80%~88%。

5．注意

乙醇和乙醚为易燃溶剂。

【思考题】

1．渗漉法的特点和适用范围是什么？

2．以醇为溶媒制备酊剂时应注意什么？

3．为何要用10~20目姜粉？

4．药粉装入渗漉器前为何要先用溶媒浸润并放置一段时间？

5．药粉装入渗漉器时过松或过紧会对浸出效果有何影响，为什么？

6．渗漉速度为何不能太快或太慢？

7．为什么要收集初漉液？

8．《中国药典》规定如何测定酊剂中的乙醇含量？

参 考 文 献

1．国家药典委员会．中华人民共和国药典（一部）．北京：化学工业出版社．2000，附录12～13．

2．国家药典委员会．中华人民共和国药典（一部）．北京：化学工业出版社．2000，535．

Exercise 1 Tinctures

Learning objectives

Practice and learn the general process to produce tinctures by percolation method with crude drugs.

Instruction

Tinctures[1-2] are clear liquid preparations of medicinal substances macerated or dissolved in ethanol of specified concentration or made by diluting the liquid extracts.

1. The general requirements of production and storage of tinctures:

(1) Unless otherwise specified, tinctures containing poisonous or potent drugs are equivalent to 10 g of the drug in 100 ml of the tincture; most of the other tinctures represent 20 g of the drug in 100 ml of the tincture.

(2) The active principle of a tincture containing poisonous or potent drugs may be determined by an assay of its intermediate product and then the potency adjusted to produce a finished product that complies with the requirements stated in the individual monograph.

(3) Tinctures may be prepared by dissolution, dilution, maceration or percolation.

a) Dissolution or Dilution Dissolve a quantity of drug powder or dilute liquid extracts with a quantity of ethanol of specified concentration, allow to stand, filter if necessary.

b) Maceration Macerate the powder drugs with a quantity of solvent in a stoppered container for 3 ~ 5 days or a specified time, stirring or shaking occasionally. Separate out the supernatant liquid, and continue the maceration in the same way until the active principles are completely extracted. Combine the extracts and add solvent to volume as required, leave standing for 24 hours, then filter.

c) Percolation (a) Either a cylindrical or a conical percolator may be used, depending on the nature of the crude drug. (b) Macerate the powder drugs with a quantity of solvent in a sealed container for some time before the percolation takes place. (c) When an amount of the initial percolate equivalent to 85% of the crude drug in the percolator has been collected, it is set aside. The rest of the percolate should be concentrated at a low temperature and the mixed products of percolation and concentration are made up to the required volume with the solvent. Leave standing for 24 hours, then filter.

(4) Tinctures may be filtered when precipitate, stored for a long time, if the contents of alcohol and active ingredients comply with the requirement.

(5) Tinctures should be preserved in light – resistant, tightly closed containers and

stored in a cool place.

2. Tests

Content of alcohol in tinctures should be determined. (See Ch.P. Appendix.)

Tincture Zingiberis

Tincture Zingiberis[3] is a TCM preparation recorded in the Ch.P. (2000), made of dry ginger extract. Dry ginger originates from the rhizome of *Zingiber officinale* Rosc., containing 2% ~ 3.5% of essential oil.

Description A pale yellow liquor, having a pleasant odor, resembling Rhizoma Zingiberis; taste hot.

Action and Indication Stomachic and carminative

Usage and Dosage oral, 2 ~ 4 ml, 3 times a day

Storage Preserve in tightly closed containers, stored in a cool place.

Exercise materials

Instrument: beaker, percolator, filter paper, funnel

Drugs and reagents: Powder of Rhizoma Zingiberis, 90% ethanol

Exercise method

1. Formulation

Powder of Rhizoma Zingiberis	200 g
90% ethanol	Q.S
Make 1000ml	

2. Procedure

(1) Preparation of fluid extract of Zingiberis (Extractum Zingiberis Liquidum)

a) Macerate 20g dried powdered Rhizoma Zingiberis with 15ml of 90% ethanol in a sealed container for 24 hours.

b) Percolate slowly at the speed of 2 ~ 4 ml per minute per 1000 g. Collect 17 ml of the initial percolate and continue the percolation, until the percolate becomes nearly colorless and a taste of ginger becomes very slight.

c) Evaporate the successive percolate below 60℃ to a thick extract, mix with the initial percolate, and filter.

(2) Preparation of Zingiberis Tincture

Dilute 20 ml of the fluid extract of Zingiberis with 90% ethanol to 100 ml. Allow to stand until the fluid becomes clear, then filter.

3. Assay of fluid extract of Zingiberis

It contains not less than 4.5% of ether - soluble extractive (See Extractum Zingiberis

Liquidum in Ch.P.).

4. Test of Tincture Zingiberis

Ethanol content 80% ~ 88% (See Ch.P.Appendix: Determination of Ethanol).

Questions

1. What are the characters and subject range of percolation?
2. What should be paid attention to when preparing tinctures by ethanol?
3. What kind of ginger powder should be used?
4. Why should the ginger powder be macerated for 24 hours before it is packed into the percolator?
5. When putting the ginger powder into the percolator, it should be packed with uniform compactness. Why?
6. Why should the rate of percolation not be too slow or fast?
7. Why collect the initial percolate?

References

1. Pharmacopoeia Commission of PRC. Pharmacopoeia of the People's Republic of China (English edition), Vol. Ⅰ. Beijing: Chemical Industry Press. 1997, Appendix Ⅰ A-9

2. Pharmacopoeia Commission of PRC. Pharmacopoeia of the People's Republic of China (Vol. Ⅰ). Beijing: Chemical Industry Press. 2000, Appendix 12 ~ 13, 535

3. Pharmacopoeia Commission of PRC. Pharmacopoeia of the People's Republic of China (English edition) Vol. Ⅰ. Beijing: Chemical Industry Press. 1997, 277

实验二　合剂（口服液）

【实验目的】

1．熟悉中药口服液的质量要求。

2．通过口服液的制备练习，掌握中药口服液的一般制法。

【实验指导】

合剂[1]是指药材用水或其他溶剂，采用适宜方法提取、纯化、浓缩制成的内服液体制剂。单剂量包装者习称“口服液”。

1．制备中药口服液的一般要求

口服液在生产与贮藏期间应符合下列有关规定：

（1）一般情况下，制备口服液的药材应洗净，适当加工成片、段或粗粉，按规定的方法提取，纯化，浓缩到规定的相对密度；含有挥发性成分的药材宜先提取挥发性成分，再与余药共同煎煮。

（2）口服液应在清洁避菌的环境中配制，及时灌装于无菌的洁净干燥容器中。

（3）口服液中可加入适宜的附加剂，其品种与用量应符合国家标准的有关规定，不得影响制品的稳定性，应避免对检验产生干扰。必要时亦可加入适量的乙醇。

（4）口服液若加蔗糖作为附加剂，除另有规定外，其含蔗糖量不高于20%（g/ml）。

（5）另有规定外，口服液应澄清。不得有酸败、异臭、产生气体或其他变质现象。

（6）合剂应密封，置阴凉处贮藏。在贮藏期间允许有少量轻摇易散的沉淀。

2．口服液的适口性

除了以上对口服液的要求以外，口服液体制剂的适口性也是生产上值得考虑的重要因素，关系到病人的可接受性或依从性问题。虽然传统上有“苦口良药”的说法，但是现在病人实际上希望口服的药液有好的口感或者最起码能够忍受其气味，特别是对于儿童和老人。

适口性受到感觉的综合影响，包括味觉和嗅觉。产品的构成、外观和温度对感觉也是有影响的。例如，含有沙砾的液体病人是不大愿意服用的。化合物的结构与其气味是相关联的。低分子量的盐倾向于咸，而高分子量的盐倾向于苦。含氮化合物一般倾向于特别苦，例如生物碱。含羟基的小分子化合物，随着羟基数量的增加，会增加甜度。小分子有机酯、醇、醛可能有令人愉快的气味，并且由于挥发作用有清凉的感觉。某些特殊结构的化合物具有非常的甜度，已经开发成甜味剂。

适合掩盖不良气味的调味剂常常是通过体验来发现的。在本次实验中，指导教师可以推荐几种调味剂供学生来调整原有的口服液气味。

3．口服液的检查

（1）一般应制定相对密度、pH值等检查项目。

（2）装量和装量检查　检查法　取供试品5支，将内容物分别倒入经校正的干燥量筒内，在室温下检视，每支装量与标示装量相比较，少于标示装量的不得多于 1 支，并不得少于标示装量的 95%。

（3）微生物限量　应符合有关规定（参见《中华人民共和国药典》附录）。

实验　清热解毒口服液

清热解毒口服液（Qingre Jiedu Koufuye）是《中华人民共和国药典》收载的中药制剂[2]。

本品为中药复方制成的口服液，以绿原酸和栀子苷作本制剂的标志性定性成分，黄芩苷作为定量指标。

性状：本品为棕红色的液体；味甜、微苦。

功能与主治：清热解毒。用于热毒壅盛所致发热面赤，烦躁口渴，咽喉肿痛等症；流感、上呼吸道感染见上述证候者。

用法用量：口服，一次 10～20ml，一日 3 次；或遵医嘱。

规格：每支装 10ml

贮藏：密封，置阴凉处。

【实验材料】

仪器：天平、烧杯 1000ml、量筒（1000ml、100ml）、玻璃漏斗（9cm、4cm）、布氏漏斗（7cm）、比重瓶、冰箱、易拉瓶、封口机、灭菌锅、水浴、蒸发皿、容量瓶（100ml、1ml）、微量注射器、紫外分析仪、pH 计、电炉、高效液相色谱仪、色谱柱（十八烷基硅烷键合硅胶为填充剂）、分析天平、减压干燥器等。

药品和试剂：石膏、金银花、玄参、地黄、连翘、栀子、甜地丁、黄芩、龙胆、板蓝根、知母、麦冬、乙醇、活性炭、蒸馏水、硅胶 G 薄层板、醋酸丁酯、甲酸、氯仿、丙酮、50%硫酸乙醇液、磷酸、绿原酸、栀子苷、黄芩苷等。

【实验方法】

1．处方

石膏 670g	金银花 134g	玄参 107g	地黄 80g
连翘 67g	栀子 67g	甜地丁 67g	黄芩 67g
龙胆 67g	板蓝根 67g	知母 54g	麦冬 54g
蒸馏水适量			制成 1000ml

（学生实验用十分之一量）

2．制法

（1）提取　以上十二味，除金银花、黄芩外，取其余生石膏等十味先加适量水温浸 1 小时，煎煮二次（待沸腾后，稍冷加金银花和黄芩），第一次 1 小时，第二次 40 分钟，滤过，合并滤液，滤液浓缩到相对密度约为 1.2。

（2）精制　在上述浓缩液中加入乙醇，使含醇量达 65%～70%，冷藏 48 小时，滤过，回收乙醇得浓缩液。

（3）配液　在上述浓缩液中加蒸馏水至100ml，加入0.5%活性炭，加热30分钟，滤过，加水到100ml，滤过，得药液。

（4）灌封和灭菌　将上述精制过的药液分装于10ml易拉瓶中，以流通蒸汽或煮沸30分钟，即得成品。

3．鉴别和检查

（1）取本品10ml，置水浴上蒸干，残渣加乙醇5ml使溶解，滤过，滤液浓缩至2ml，作为供试品溶液。另取绿原酸对照品，加乙醇制成每1ml含1mg的溶液，作为对照品溶液。照薄层色谱法（参照《中华人民共和国药典》（一部）附录）试验，吸取上述两种溶液各10μl，分别点于同一硅胶G薄层板上，以醋酸丁酯－甲酸－水（14∶5∶5）上层溶液为展开剂，展开，取出，晾干，在紫外光灯（365nm）下检视。供试品色谱中，在与对照品色谱相应的位置上，显相同颜色的荧光斑点。

（2）取本品10ml，置水浴上蒸干，残渣加丙酮2ml使溶解，取上清液作为供试品溶液。另取栀子苷对照品，加丙酮制成每1ml含0.5mg的溶液，作为对照品溶液。照薄层色谱法（参照《中华人民共和国药典》（一部）附录）试验，吸取上述两种溶液各10μl，分别点于同一硅胶G薄层板上，以氯仿－甲醇（3∶1）为展开剂，展开，取出，晾干，喷以50%硫酸乙醇溶液，于100℃加热至斑点显色清晰。供试品色谱中，在与对照品色谱相应的位置上，显相同颜色的荧光斑点。

（3）pH值　应为4.5～6.5。

（4）含量测定　照高效液相色谱法（参照《中华人民共和国药典》（一部）附录）测定。

色谱条件与系统适用性试验　用十八烷键合硅胶为填充剂；甲醇－水－磷酸（50∶50∶0.3）为流动相；检测波长为276nm。理论板数按黄芩苷峰计算应不低于1000。

对照品溶液的制备　精密称取在100℃减压干燥至恒重的黄芩苷对照品，加乙醇制成每1ml含0.01mg的溶液，作为对照品溶液。

供试品溶液的制备　精密量取装量项下的本品2ml，置100ml量瓶中，加乙醇适量，振摇，用乙醇稀释至刻度，摇匀，放置，滤过，取续滤液作为供试品溶液。

测定法　分别精密吸取对照品溶液与供试品溶液各10μl，注入液相色谱仪，测定，即得。

本品每支含黄芩按黄芩苷（$C_{21}H_{18}O_{11}$）计，不得少于10.0mg。

实验　银黄口服液

银黄口服液（Yinhuang Koufuye）是《中华人民共和国药典》（一部）收载的中药口服制剂[3]。本品为金银花提取物与黄芩提取物制成的口服液。本品每支含金银花提取物以绿原酸（$C_{16}H_{18}O_9$）计，不得少于0.108g；含黄芩提取物以黄芩苷（$C_{21}H_{18}O_{11}$）计，不得少于0.216g。

性状：本品为红棕色的澄清液体；味甜、微苦。

功能与主治：清热解毒，消炎。用于上呼吸道感染，急性扁桃体炎，咽炎。

用法与用量：口服，一次10～20ml，一日3次；小儿酌减。

规格：每支 10ml

贮藏：密封，置阴凉处。

【实验材料】

仪器：量筒（100ml）、烧杯（100ml）、天平、pH 计、布氏漏斗（7cm）、滤纸（7cm）、电炉、易拉瓶、灭菌锅、试管、比重瓶、吸量管（2ml）、容量瓶（100ml）、紫外分光光度计等。

药品和试剂：金银花提取物、黄芩提取物、氢氧化钠、单糖浆、蒸馏水、硝酸钠、硝酸铝、二氯氧化锆、盐酸等。

【实验方法】

1．处方

金银花提取物（以绿原酸计）	12g
黄芩提取物（以黄芩苷计）	24g
注射用水加至	1000ml

（学生实验用十分之一量）

2．制法

（1）溶解　取金银花提取物加水适量使溶解。黄芩提取物加适量水使溶解，再用 8% 氢氧化钠溶液调节 pH 值至 8，滤过。

（2）调配　将黄芩提取物溶液与金银花提取物溶液合并，用 8% 氢氧化钠溶液调节 pH 至 7.2，煮沸 1 小时，滤过，加入单糖浆或其他调味剂适量，加水至近全量，搅匀，用 8% 氢氧化钠溶液调节 pH 至 7.2，加水至 100ml，滤过。

（3）灌封和灭菌　灌封于 10ml 易拉瓶中，以流通蒸汽灭菌 30 分钟，即得。

3．鉴别和检查

（1）取本品 1ml，加 5% 硝酸钠溶液与 10% 硝酸铝溶液各 0.3ml，生成黄色沉淀；再加 5% 氢氧化钠溶液使成碱性，沉淀即溶解，溶液显棕红色。

（2）取本品 0.1ml，加水 10ml，摇匀，取溶液 2ml，加 5% 二氯氧化锆溶液 1～2 滴，溶液显黄色，再加盐酸 1～2 滴，黄色不褪。

（3）相对密度　应不低于 1.05（参见《中国药典》附录）。

（4）pH 值　应为 5.5～7.0（参见《中国药典》附录）。

（5）其他　应符合合剂有关的各项规定（参见《中国药典》附录）。

（6）评价口服液的适口性。

4．含量测定

精密量取本品 2ml，置 100ml 量瓶中，加水至刻度，摇匀，精密量取 2ml，置 100ml 量瓶中，加 0.2mol/L 盐酸溶液至刻度，摇匀，照分光光度法（《中国药典》附录ⅤA），在 278nm 与 318nm 的波长处分别测定吸收度，按下式计算，即得。

$$c_1 = 2.599 \times E_{318} - 1.522 \times E_{278}$$

$$c_1 = 2.121 \times E_{278} - 1 - 0.9169 \times E_{318}$$

$$绿原酸（C_{16}H_{18}O_9）的含量（mg/ml）= \frac{c_1 \times 100 \times 100}{100 \times 2 \times 2}$$

$$黄芩苷（C_{21}H_{18}O_{11}）的含量（mg/ml）= \frac{c_2 \times 100 \times 100}{100 \times 2 \times 2}$$

式中　c_1 为供试品溶液中绿原酸浓度，mg/100ml；

c_2 为供试品溶液中黄芩苷浓度，mg/100ml；

E_{278}为供试品溶液在 278nm 波长处测得的吸收度；

E_{318}为供试品溶液在 318nm 波长处测得的吸收度。

【思考题】

1．金银花提取物、黄芩提取物是如何制备的？
2．在溶解黄芩提取物时加碱的目的是什么？
3．制备口服液的基本要求和关键步骤是什么？
4．口服液成分的气味如何？

参　考　文　献

1．国家药典委员会．中华人民共和国药典（一部）．北京：化学工业出版社．2000，附录 11．
2．国家药典委员会．中华人民共和国药典（一部）．北京：化学工业出版社．2000，592
3．国家药典委员会．中华人民共和国药典（一部）．北京：化学工业出版社．2000，580

Exercise 2 Mixtures (Oral Liquids)

Exercise objectives

1. Understand the quality control of oral liquids of the Traditional Chinese Medicine.

2. Grasp the general preparation method of oral liquids of the Traditional Chinese Medicine by exercise of preparing mixtures.

Instruction

Mixtures[1] are liquid preparations intended for oral administration, prepared by extracting the crude drugs with water or other solvents in suitable ways, purifying and concentrating the extracts. Oral liquid is a more popular name for single – dose mixture.

1. General requirements for preparation of mixtures

(1) Unless specified otherwise, the crude drugs should be washed clean, and processed to slices, sections or coarse powder, extracted, purified and concentrated to specified relative density by a method. The volatile ingredients in crude drugs should be extracted at first, then the crude drugs remaining decocted with the other drugs together.

(2) Mixtures should be prepared under clean aseptic circumstances, and filled in sterile, clean and dry containers.

(3) Suitable additives may be added to mixtures. The variety and quantity to be used should comply with the requirements of the national standard and must not affect the stability or interfere with the tests for mixtures. If necessary, mixtures could also contain a proper quantity of alcohol.

(4) If sucrose is used as an additive in mixtures, the content of it should not be more than 20% (g/g).

(5) Mixtures should not become rancid, produce abnormal odours or gas, and must not have deteriorated.

(6) Mixtures should be preserved in tightly closed containers and stored in a cool and dry place. Mixtures are allowed to have small amount of dispersible precipitates during storage.

2. Palatability of oral liquids

Palatability must be considered in producing an oral liquid product, that is an important determinant of patient acceptance or compliance with oral liquid dosage forms, besides the above requirement of oral liquids. Although "the worse the taste of the medication, the better the cure" was traditionally the prevailing attitude, actually patients now expect oral liquid medications that are pleasantly, or at least tolerably, flavored. This is especially true with children and older adults.

Palatability is influenced by a combination of sensory perceptions including taste and smell. Texture, appearance, and temperature of the products also influences sensory perceptions. For example, a gritty liquid is poorly received to take orally by patients. There is a correlation between the chemical structure of a compound and its taste and smell. Low molecular weight salts tend to taste salty, but higher molecular weight salts tend toward bitterness. Nitrogen containing compounds, such as the alkaloids, usually tend to be quite bitter. Small organic compounds containing hydroxyl groups tend to become increasingly sweet as the number of OH groups increase. Organic esters, alcohols, and aldehydes with low molecular weight may have pleasant taste and cool sensation produced by their volatility. Some compounds with special structure are very sweet and have been developed as sweeteners.

Discovering the flavoring agent best suited to masking an unpleasant taste is often a empirical matter. In this exercise, instructors may recommend some flavoring agents for students to mask the given taste of oral liquids.

3. Tests

(1) In general, relative density and pH value etc. should be determined.

(2) Content variation For mixtures packed in a single dose, the content variation should be examined.

Procedure Take 5 bottles of a mixture, pour the content separately to the calibrated dry graduated cylinders, and examine at room temperature. Compare the filling volume of each pack with the labelled amount: the content of not more than 1 bottle may be less than the labelled amount, and none may be less than 95% of the labelled amount.

Mixtures comply with the requirements stated in Minimum Fill (Ch.P. Appendix).

(3) Microbial limit test Comply with the requirements stated under Microbial Limit Test (Ch.P. Appendix).

Qingre Jiedu Oral Liquid (Qingre Jiedu Koufuye)

Qingre Jiedu Koufuye[2] is an oral liquid of traditional Chinese medicine recorded in the Pharmacopeia of the People's Republic of China. Chlorogenic acid and geniposide are the marker ingredients for identification of the preparation, and baicalin as an active ingredient should be assayed.

Description A brownish-red liquid; taste is sweet, slightly bitter.

Action To remove heat and counteract toxicity.

Indication Influenza, infection of upper respiratory tract and different febrile diseases.

Usage and Dosage 10 ~ 20 ml, 3 times a day; or follow physician's advice.

Specification 10 ml per ampoule

Storage Preserve in tightly closed containers, stored in a cool place.

Exercise materials

Instrument: balance, beaker (1000ml), graduated cylinder (1000ml、100ml), glass funnel (9cm, 4cm), Buchner funnel (7cm), filter paper (7cm), density bottle, refrigerator, phial, sealing machine, sterilizing kettle, water bath, evaporating dish, volumetric flask (100ml, 1ml), micro – syringe, UV spectrophotometer, pH meter, hotplate, HPLC unit, chromatographic column (ODS C – 18), analytical balance, and vacuum oven, etc.

Drugs and reagents: Gypsum Fibrosum, Flos Lonicerae, Radix Scrophulariae, Radix Rehmanniae, Fructus Forsythiae, Fructus Gardeniae, Herba Gueldenstaedtiae, Radix Scutellariae, Radix Gentianae, Radix Isatidis, Rhizoma Anemarrhenae, Radix Ophiopogonis, ethanol, active charcoal, distilled water, silica gel G plate, ethyl acetate, formic acid, chloroform, acetone, 50% sulfuric acid solution in ethanol, phosphoric acid, fluorescent, chlorogenic acid, geniposide, and baicalin, etc.

Exercise methods

1. Formulation

Gypsum Fibrosum 670g; Flos Lonicerae 134g; Radix Scrophulariae 107g; Radix Rehmanniae 80g; Fructus Forsythiae 670g; Fructus Gardeniae 670g; Herba Gueldenstaedtiae 670g; Radix Scutellariae 67g; Radix Gentianae 67g; Radix Isatidis 67g; Rhizoma Anemarrhenae 54g; Radix Ophiopogonis 54g.

Distilled water q.s. to 1000ml

Tenth for the student's exercise

2. Procedure

(1) Extraction Warmly macerate Gypsum Fibrosum and other ingredients, except Flos Lonicerae and Radix Scutellariae, with water for 1 hour, decoct twice (after boiling, allow to cool slightly, add Flos Lonicerae and Radix Scutellariae), 1 hour for the first time, 40 minutes for the second time, filter. Combine the filtrates and concentrate to a thin extract with a relative density of about 1. 17.

(2) Purification To add ethanol to a content of 65% ~ 70% ethanol, store at a lower temperature for 48 hours, filter. Recover ethanol.

(3) Preparation To add 0.5% quantity of active charcoal, heat for 30 minutes and filter. Add water to a volume of 1000 ml, filter, pack and sterilize.

3. Identification

(1) Evaporate 10ml on a water bath until dry, dissolve the residue in 5ml of ethanol, filter and concentrate the filtrate to about 2 ml as the test solution. Dissolve chlorogenic acid CRS in ethanol to produce a solution containing 1 mg per ml as the reference solution. Carry out the method for thin layer chromatography (Ch.P.Appendix Ⅵ B), using silica gel G as the coating substance and the upper layer of ethyl acetate – formic acid – water (14:5:5) as the mobile phase. Apply 10 μl each of the two solutions separately to the plate. After developing and removal of the plate and dry it in air, examine under ultraviolet light (365 nm), the fluorescent spot in the chromatogram obtained with the test solution corresponds in position and colour to the spot in the chromatogram obtained with the reference solution.

(2) Evaporate 10 ml of the mixture on a water bath to dryness, dissolve the residue in 2 ml of acetone, use the supernatant as the test solution. Dissolve geniposide CRS in acetone to produce a solution containing 0.5 mg per ml as the reference solution. Carry out the method for thin layer chromatography (Ch.P.Appendix VI B), using silica gel G as the coating substance and a mixture of chloroform – methanol (3:1) as the mobile phase. Apply 10 ml of each of the two solutions separately to the plate. After developing and removal of the plate and dry it in air, spray with 50% sulfuric acid solution in ethanol, heat at 100℃ to visualize the spots clearly. The spot in the chromatogram obtained with the test solution corresponds in position and colour to the spot in the chromatogram obtained with the reference solution.

(3) pH value 4.5 ~ 6.5 (Appendix Ⅶ G).

4. Assay

Carry out the method of high performance liquid chromatography (Ch.P.Appendix).

Chromatographic system and system suitability: Use octadecylsilance bonded silica gel as the stationary phase and a mixture of methanol – water – phosphoric acid (50:50:0.3) as the mobile phase. The wavelength of the detector is 276 nm. The number of theoretical plates of the column is not less than 1000, calculated with the reference to the peak of baicalin.

Preparation of the reference solution: Weigh accurately a quantity of baicalin CRS, dried to constant weight at 100℃ in vacuum, dissolve in ethanol to produce a solution containing 0.01 mg per ml as the reference solution.

Preparation of the test solution: Measure accurately 2 ml, obtained under the test of packing variation, to a 100 ml volumetric flask, add a quantity of ethanol, shake well, dilute with ethanol to the volume, shake well, allow to stand, filter and use the successive filtrate as the test solution.

Procedure Inject accurately 10 μl each of the reference solution and the test solution into the column, respectively, and determine.

It contains not less than 10.0 mg of baicalin ($C_{21}H_{18}O_{11}$) per phial, referred to Radix Scutellariae.

Yinhuang Oral Liquid (Yinhuang Koufuye)

Yinhuang Koufuye[3] is an oral preparation of TCM recorded in the Pharmacopeia of the People's republic of China. The mixture is made – up with Extractum Lonicerae and Extractum Scutellariae. It contains not less than 0.108 g of chlorogenic acid ($C_{16}H_{18}O_9$) per vial, referred to Extractum Lonicerae; not less than 0.216 g of baicalin ($C_{21}H_{18}O_{11}$) per vial, referred to Extractum Scutellariae.

Description A clear reddish – brown liquid; taste is sweet, slightly bitter.

Action To remove heat and toxicity, to diminish inflammation.

Indication Infection of upper respiratory tract, acute tonsillitis, pharyngitis.

Usage and dosage 10 ~ 20ml, 3 times a day; appropriate reduction of the dosage for children.

Specification 10ml per vial.

Storage Preserve in tightly closed containers, stored in a cool place.

Exercise materials

Instruments: graduated cylinder (100ml), beaker (100ml), balance, pH meter, Buchner funnel (7cm), filter paper (7cm), electric hot plate, phial, sterilizing kettle, test tube, density bottle, buret (2ml)、volumetric flask (100ml), and UV spectrophotometer, etc.

Drugs and reagents: extractum lonicerae, extractum scutellariae, sodium hydroxide, syrup, distilled water, sodium nitrate, aluminium nitrate, zirconium oxychloride, hydrochloric acid, chlorogenic acid, and baicalin, etc.

Exercise methods

1. Formulation

Extractum Lonicerae 12g (calculated as chlorogenic acid);

Extractum Scutellariae 24g (calculated as baicalin).

Distilled water ad. 1000ml

Tenth for the student's exercise.

2. Procedure

(1) Dissolve Dissolve the above two ingredients with water respectively. Add 8% solution of sodium hydroxide to the dissolved Extractum Scutellariae to adjust to pH 8, and filter.

(2) Preparation Combine the filtrate of solution of Extractum Scutellariae with the solution of Extractum Lonicerae, then adjust to pH 7.2 by adding 8% solution of sodium hydroxide, decoct for 1 hour and filter, add a quantity of flavoring agents (Syrups Simplex or others) to the filtrate and dilute with water to almost the total amount, mix well, adjust to pH 7.2 with 8% sodium hydroxide, dilute with water to 100 ml, filter, pack, seal and sterilize.

3. Identification

(1) To 1 ml of the mixture add 0.3 ml of a 5% solution of sodium nitrate and a 10% sodium of aluminium nitrate separately; a yellow precipitate is produced. Add a 5% solution of sodium hydroxide to adjust to alkaline, the precipitate is dissolved and the solution turns to brown – red colour.

(2) To 0.1 ml of the mixture add 10 ml of water, mix well, to 2 ml of the solution add 1 ~ 2 drops of a 5% solution of zirconium oxychloride; a yellow colour is produced and add 1 ~ 2 drops of hydrochloric acid, the colour is unchanged.

(3) Relate density Not less than 1.05 (Ch.P.Appendix).

(4) pH value 5.5 ~ 7.0 (Ch.P.Appendix).

(5) Other requirements Complies with the general requirements for mixtures (Ch. P.Appendix).

(6) Assess palatability of oral liquids

4. Assay

Measure accurately 2 ml of the mixture in a 100 ml volumetric flask, dilute with water to volume and mix well. Transfer accurately 2 ml to a 100 ml volumetric flask, add 0.2mol/L hydrochloric acid solution to volume, and mix well. Carry out the method for spectrophotometry (Ch.P.Appendix V A), measure the absorbance at 278 and 318 nm, calculate the content from the following expression.

$$c_1 = 2.599 \times A_{318} - 1.522 \times A_{278}$$

$$c_1 = 2.121 \times A_{278} - 1 - 0.9169 \times A_{318}$$

$$\text{chlorogenic acid } (C_{16}H_{18}O_9) \text{ (mg/ml)} = \frac{c_1 \times 100 \times 100}{100 \times 2 \times 2}$$

$$\text{baicalin } (C_{21}H_{18}O_{11}) \text{ (mg/ml)} = \frac{c_2 \times 100 \times 100}{100 \times 2 \times 2}$$

where c_1 is concentration of chlorogenic acid in the test solution;

c_2 is concentration of baicalin in the test solution;

A_{278} is absorbance of the test solution at 278 nm;

A_{318} is absorbance of the test solution at 318 nm;

It contains not less than 0.108 g of chlorogenic acid ($C_{16}H_{18}O_9$) per vial, referred to Extractum Lonicerae; not less than 0.216 g of baicalin ($C_{21}H_{18}O_{11}$) per vial, referred to

Extractum Scutellariae.

Questions

1. What are the principal constituents of Flos Lonicerae, Fructus Gardeniae, and Radix Scutellariae?

2. Why is a solution of sodium hydroxide added for dissolving extractum scutellariae?

3. What are the essential demands and key steps of preparing the oral liquid?

4. How are the taste and smell of the herb ingredients in the mixtures?

Reference

1. Pharmacopoeia Commission of PRC. Pharmacopoeia of the People's Republic of China (English Edition. Volume Ⅰ). Beijing: Chemical Industry Press. 1997, 415, Appendix A-8.

2. Pharmacopoeia Commission of PRC. Pharmacopoeia of the People's Republic of China (English Edition. Volume Ⅰ), Beijing: Chemical Industry Press, 1997, 342.

3. Pharmacopoeia Commission of PRC. Pharmacopoeia of the People's Republic of China (English Edition. Volume Ⅰ), Beijing: Chemical Industry Press, 1997, 423.

实验三　注　射　剂

【实验目的】

1．熟悉中药注射剂的质量要求。

2．通过黄芪注射液的制备，掌握中草药注射剂的一般制法。

【实验指导】

中药或天然药物注射剂[1]是指药材中提取的药用物质，经由合适的方法制成的可供注入体内使用的灭菌溶液、混悬液和乳液，以及供临用前配制成注射溶液的灭菌粉末或浓缩液。注射剂分为注射液、注射用无菌粉末和注射用无菌浓溶液。

1．中药或天然药物注射剂的一般要求

（1）除非特殊情况，一般药材须用一种合适的方法经过提取和精制得到半成品，然后用于制备注射剂。

（2）注射剂所用的溶剂应该是安全无害的，对治疗效果和药品质量无不良影响。注射用溶剂分为两类：水性溶剂和非水溶剂。

最常用的水性溶剂为注射用水，亦可用0.9%氯化钠注射液或其他适宜的水溶液。通常非水性溶剂为植物油，主要为豆油，应符合注射用油要求。乙醇、丙二醇、聚乙二醇的水溶液等也用作注射溶剂。

（3）供静脉和输液用的注射剂为无菌水溶液或水作为连续相的乳浊液。除了一般的要求外，该类注射剂不应含有微生物和热原，应符合中国药典规定的草酸盐、钾离子、颗粒和溶血检查的要求，并且尽可能的与血液等渗。供静脉注射的乳液中的分散液滴的大小一般应小于1μm。乳液可以用高压灭菌器灭菌，贮藏时保持稳定。乳液不得用于脊髓内给药。

（4）供直接分装成注射用无菌粉末的原料药应无菌，凡用冷冻干燥法者，其药液应无菌，灌装时装量差异应控制在±4%以内。供静脉注射的粉末应无菌，并且不应含有微生物和热原，应符合中国药典规定的草酸盐、钾离子、颗粒和溶血检查的要求。临用前制备药液的方法应在标签上写明。应用合适的溶剂在使用前将粉末溶解。“注射用”作为前缀置于药名之前。

（5）除另有规定外，注射用混悬液中药物的细度应控制在15μm以下，15~20μm（间有个别20~50μm）者不得超过10%。

（6）配制注射剂时，可按药物的性质加入适宜的附加剂。附加剂有渗透压调节剂、pH值调节剂、增溶剂、抗氧剂以及抑菌剂等。附加剂如为抑菌剂时，用量应能抑制注射液内微生物的生长。常用的抑菌剂与用量（g/ml）为0.5%苯酚，0.3%甲酚，0.5%三氯叔丁醇等。加有抑菌剂的注射液，仍应用适宜的方法灭菌。注射量超过5ml的注射液，添加的抑菌剂必须特别审慎选择。供静脉（除另有规定外）或椎管注射用的注射液，不得添加抑菌剂，使用增溶剂也应慎重。供椎管注射用的注射液，不得加入任何抑菌剂和增溶剂。加有抑菌剂的注射剂，应在标签上说明所加抑菌剂的名称与浓度。

(7) 灌装注射剂的容器有玻璃安瓿和玻璃瓶、塑料瓶或塑料袋，应符合有关国家标准。容器胶塞和塑料隔离膜应符合有关规定。

(8) 注射剂的配制应使用洁净、干燥、无菌的容器。配制注射用油溶液时，应先将精制的油在150℃干热灭菌1~2小时，并放冷至适宜的温度备用。注射剂在配制过程中，应严密防止变质与污染微生物、热原等。已调配的药液应在当日内完成灌封、灭菌。如不能在当日内完成，必须将药液在不变质与不易繁殖微生物的条件下保存；供静脉及椎管注射用的注射剂，更应严格控制。

(9) 药液制备好后，应迅速灌装。接触空气易变质的药物，在灌装过程中，容器内应排除空气，填充二氧化碳或氮等气体后熔封。

(10) 注射剂密封后，可根据药物的性质选用适宜的方法灭菌，必须保证成品无菌。

(11) 熔封的注射剂在灭菌时或灭菌后，应采用减压法或其他适宜的方法进行容器检漏。

(12) 注射剂应根据药品的稳定性，选择适合的条件贮藏。

2．过滤设备

在注射剂生产中常用垂熔玻璃滤器、砂滤棒、板框压滤机和膜滤器等。

(1) 垂熔玻璃滤器（砂芯滤器）：系以硬质中性玻璃细粉烧结成具有一定孔径的滤器。分为垂熔玻璃漏斗、滤球和滤棒等。按滤板的孔径粗细孔径大小分为不同规格。

垂熔玻璃滤器用途说明

编号	微孔平均直径（μm）	主要用途
1	80~120	收集和扩散气体
2	40~80	滤除大颗粒之沉淀
3	15~40	滤除一般化学溶液中杂质
4	5~15	采用减压过滤方法，滤除溶液中沉淀杂质
5	2~5	采用减压过滤方法，滤除细小沉淀或较大细菌
6	小于2	采用减压过滤方法，滤除细菌

使用注意事项：

新的玻璃滤器在使用前应以热盐酸或硫酸先行抽滤，并立即用蒸馏水洗净。经过这个预处理，滤器中灰尘等的外来杂质可以除去。玻璃滤器不能用以过滤浓氢氟酸，热浓磷酸，热或冷的浓碱液，也不能用上述溶液清洗。在减压和受压的情况下使用时，滤片两面的压力差不容许超过98kPa。

玻璃砂芯滤器在使用以后，有一部分沉淀物在过滤进行时被留存在玻璃砂芯的细孔中，必须有效地给以清洗，才能继续使用。可采用水压冲洗法、减压抽洗法或化学洗涤法。

(2) 微孔滤器：系以高分子材料（如混合纤维素酯）制成的多孔性薄膜为滤过介质，孔径约14~0.025μm左右，能滤除菌，制备注射液时用此滤器。

3．灌封设备

(1) 手工灌封　手工灌封适合于注射剂的小量制备。手工灌注机构造简单，依靠两个单向活塞控制药液的容量。灌注针头一般选用较长的注射针头或用玻璃管、聚乙烯塑料管拉成。安瓿的手工熔封分为单火焰法和双火焰法。单火焰法：将安瓿拿在手中，将其颈部置于火焰上，烧熔后用镊子夹住颈部上端，拉封并圆口。双火焰法：将安瓿排列在固定槽中，将瓶颈置于两个相对的火焰下熔融、拉封。封口火焰的燃料可以用煤气、汽化汽油，同时用压缩空气或氧气助燃。

（2）灌封机　灌封机针对不同的容器有多种类型。安瓿拉丝灌封机是一种以安瓿瓶为容器灌装液体并封口的自动包装设备，广泛应用于医药企业的小容量注射剂的包装。在兽药生产、化工试剂生产中也常见使用。封口燃气可使用煤气、汽油汽化气以及石油液化气，用氧气助燃。生产能力每小时可达数千只。

4．注射剂的检查[1]

（1）注射液的装量和装量检查　灌装时，每件注射液容器的装量应略微超过标示量。增加装量，以保证足够抽取和给药用量。供多次用量的注射液，每一容器的装量不得超过10次注射量。增加的装量应能保证每次注射的标示用量。

注射剂的装量

标示装量（ml）	增加量（ml）	
	易流动液体	黏稠液体
0.5	0.10	0.12
1	0.10	0.15
2.	0.15	0.25
5.	0.30	0.50
10	0.50	0.70
20	0.60	0.90
50	1.0	1.5

检查法：注射液的标示装量为2ml或2ml以下的容器取供试品5件，2ml以上至50ml者取供试品3件，开启时注意避免损失，将内容物分别用相应体积的干燥注射器（预经标化）抽尽，在室温下检视；测定油溶液或混悬液的装量时，应先加温摇匀，再用干燥注射器抽尽，放冷至室温检视。每件容器中注射液的装量均不得少于其标示量。

（2）注射剂的其他检查　注射剂其他的检查还包括可见异物、不溶性微粒、有关物质等项目，照《中国药典》关于注射剂澄明度检查的规定检查。

实验　黄芪注射液

黄芪注射液（Huangqi Zhusheye）[2]是《中华人民共和国卫生部药品标准》收载的中药制剂。本品为中药黄芪制成的注射液。黄芪来源于豆科植物蒙古黄芪 *Astragalus membranaceus*（Fisch.）Bunge. var. *mongholicus*（Bge.）Hsiao 或膜荚黄芪 *A. membranaceus*（Fisch.）Bge.。含有皂苷、黄酮和多糖等成分。本品每1ml含黄芪甲苷不得少于0.08mg。

性状：本品为黄色或淡棕黄色的澄明液体。

功能与主治：益气养元，扶正祛邪，养心通脉，健脾利湿。用于心气虚损、血脉瘀阻之病毒性心肌炎、心功能不全及脾虚湿困之肝炎。

用法与用量：肌内注射，一次 2～4ml，一日 1～2 次。静脉滴注，一次 10～20ml，一日 1 次，或遵医嘱。

规格：每支装 2ml（相当于原药材 4g）、10ml（相当于原药材 20g）。

贮藏：遮光，密封。

【实验材料】

仪器：烧瓶（1000ml，500ml）、布氏漏斗（φ9mm）、试管（10ml）、4 号垂熔玻璃漏斗、水浴、电路、普通电炉、普通天平、灌注器（或灌封机）、硅胶 G 薄层板、毛细管点样器、层析缸、紫外灯显示器和注射剂澄明度检查装置等。

材料：黄芪、乙醇、注射用水、正丁醇、氯仿、甲醇、黄芪甲苷和 10%硫酸乙醇溶液等。

【实验方法】

1．处方

黄芪		2000g
注射用水	加至	1000ml

2．制法

（1）提取　取黄芪 100g，加水适量煎煮三次，每次 1.5 小时，合并煎液，滤过，滤液浓缩至每 1ml 约相当于原药材 1～2g。

（2）精制　将浓缩液用乙醇沉淀处理二次，第一次溶液中含乙醇量为 75%，冷藏放置，过滤，回收滤液乙醇至 40ml，再加乙醇至乙醇量为 85%，冷藏放置，过滤，回收滤液乙醇并浓缩至每 1ml 相当于原药材 10g。

（3）配液　用注射用水稀释精制浓缩液至每 1ml 相当于原药材 0.75～1g，冷藏放置 12 小时，滤过，滤液浓缩至每 1ml 相当于原药材 5～6g，放冷，用 20%氢氧化钠溶液调节 pH 值至 7.5，煮沸，加入 0.125%的活性炭，煮沸 5 分钟，趁热滤过，加注射用水使成 50ml，滤过，再用 20%氢氧化钠溶液调节 pH 值至 7.5，用垂熔玻璃漏斗滤过。

（4）灌封和灭菌　手工或用灌封机灌封于 2ml 安瓿，以流通蒸气灭菌 30 分钟，即得。

3．鉴别和检查

（1）依法进行可见异物检查。

（2）取本品 1.5ml，加水至 30ml，用水饱和的正丁醇提取 2 次，每次 20ml，合并正丁醇液，用水洗涤 2 次，每次 20ml，弃去水液，正丁醇液置水浴上蒸干，残渣加甲醇 0.5ml 使溶解，作为供试品溶液．另取黄芪甲苷对照品，加甲醇制成每 1ml 含 1mg 的溶液，作为对照品溶液。照中国药典薄层色谱法（附录ⅥB）试验，吸取上述两种溶液各 2μl，分别点于同一硅胶 G 薄层板上，以氯仿－甲醇－水（13∶7∶2）10℃以下放置分层的下层溶液为展开剂，展开，取出，晾干，喷以 10%硫酸乙醇溶液，在 105℃烘至斑点显色清晰，分别置日光和紫外光灯（365nm）下检视。供试品色谱中，在与对照品色谱相应的位置上，日光下显相同的棕褐色斑点，紫外光灯（365nm）下显相同的橙黄色荧光斑点。

【思考题】

1．黄芪的主要有效成分是什么？

2．制备注射剂的基本要求是什么？

3．制备黄芪注射液的各步骤的目的是什么？

参 考 文 献

1．中国国家药典委员会．中华人民共和国药典（一部）．北京：化学工业出版社．2000，附录16

2．中华人民共和国卫生部．中华人民共和国卫生部药品标准：中药成方制剂十七分册．北京：人民卫生出版社．1998，256

Exercise 3 Injection

Learning Objectives

Following study of the topic of parenteral solutions, the student should be able to:

1. Understand special requirements for control of the quality of TCM injections.
2. Practice and understand the general method for preparation of herbal injections.

Instruction

Injections of traditional Chinese medicines or natural medicinal products are sterile products containing drug substances extracted from crude drugs, intended for parenteral administration into the human body, including solutions, suspension or emulsions, as well as sterile powders or liquid concentrates, which, on the addition of suitable solvents, yield solution before use. They can be divided into injections, sterile powders for injection, and sterile concentrated liguids for injection.

1. General requirements for production of injections of traditional Chinese medicines and natural medicinal products

(1) Unless specified otherwise, crude drugs are extracted and purified using available methods to produce the intermediate products which are put into the manufacture of injections.

(2) Solvents Solvents employed for injections are safe and harmless, and have no effect on therapeutic efficiency and quality of the drug. Solvents for injections are classified into two kinds: aqueous and nonaqueous solvents. They should meet the following requirements.

Aqueous solvents: Water for injection is the most commonly used aqueous solvent, and aqueous solution of 0.9% of sodium chloride or other appropriate substances may also be employed.

Nonaqueous solvents: Nonaqueous solvents commonly employed are vegetable oils mainly being bean oil which meets the requirements of bean oil for injection. In addition, the aqueous solutions such as alcohol, propylene glycol, polyethylene glycol etc. may also be applied.

(3) Injections for intravenous and infusing use Injections for intravenous and infusing use are sterile aqueous solutions or emulsions in which water acts as the continuous phase. In addition to general requirements, these kinds of injections should be free from microbiological organisms and pyrogens, and comply with tests for oxalates, potassium ion, particulate matter and haemolysis and so on. They are made iso – osmotic with blood as far as possible. The bulk of the dispersed particulates of emulsions for intravenous use should be

less than 1 μm in size. The emulsions may be sterilized using autoclave and are stable for storage. They are not allowed to be administered for intraspinal route.

(4) Powders for injections The raw material to be distributed to the final containers should be sterile. Where powders for injections are prepared by lyophilization, the solution of medicaments used must be sterile, and the volume filled in each container must not deviate from the nominal volume exceeding ±4%. Powders for intravenous injection should be sterile and free from microbiological organisms and pyrogens, comply with tests for oxalated, potassium ion, particulate matter and haemolysis and so on. The procedures of preparing solution before use are designated on labels.

Where powders need to dissolve in suitable solvents before use, the term of "for injection" is prefixed to the names of medicaments.

(5) Additives Where injections are produced, suitable additives may be added, depending upon the characteristics of the medicaments. Additives are generally composed of osmotic adjustors, adjustors for pH values, solubilizing agents, antioxidants and bacteriostatic agents and so on. Antioxidants contain sodium sulphite, bisulphate, metabisulphite and cysteine and so on. Bacteriostatic agents are added in the concentrations that will prohibit the growth of microorganisms in the injections. Variety and concentration (g/ml) of bacteriostatic agents commonly used are phenol 0.5%, cresol 0.3%, tert – trichlorobutyl alcohol 0.5% and so on. Sterilization processes are still required even though bacteriostatic agents applied. Where injections are to be used in volume exceeding 5ml, the bacteriostatic agents should be selected with special caution. Unless specified otherwise, no bacteriostatic agents are added to injections for intravenous administration, and caution should be taken in use of solubilizing agents for this purpose. For injections for intraspinal routes, neither of the additives is allowed.

(6) Containers Unless specified otherwise, containers to be filled with injections, involving glass ampoules and vials, plastic vials or bags should comply with the requirements of national standards. The rubber closures and the isolating plastic membranes should also comply with the related specifications. The name and concentration of the bacteriostatic agent added in an injection should be shown on the label of the injection.

(7) Production Production of injections should follow the procedures concerned and use clean, dry and sterilized containers.

In production of oil solutions, refined oil should be previously heat – sterilized at a temperature of 150℃ for 1 ~ 2 hours, then allowed to cool to an appropriate temperature for use.

During the manufacturing of injections, effective measures should be adopted to avoid the microbial contamination and to prevent deterioration. The preparation of the medicament solution, filling, sealing and sterilization should be completed within one day. If not, the solution of medicaments should be preserved under aseptic condition to prevent deterioration and the growth of microorganisms. This is important for injections, in particular, intended for administration by intravenous or intraspinal routes.

(8) Filling The solution of medicaments having been prepared should be filled promptly. For solutions containing medicaments liable to deterioration on exposure to air, the air in the containers should be excluded or displaced by inert gases such as carbon dioxide or nitrogen in the process of filling before the containers are sealed by fusion.

(9) Sterilization After being closed hermetically, injections are sterilized using the appropriate methods according to the characteristics of the medicaments to ensure to sterility of the finished products.

(10) Leak – proof After being sealed by fusion, containers of injections should undergo leak – proof test under reduced pressure or by other suitable methods during or after the sterilizing process.

(11) Storage The storage of injections complies with the related requirements according to their stability.

2. Tests

(1) Volume of injection Each container of on injection is filled with a volume in slight excess of the labeled quantity. The excess quantities are usually sufficient to permit withdraw and administration of the labeled quantity. A container may contain medicaments of multiple doses, but not more than 10 doses, and the excess quantity in such containers is sufficient to permit withdraw and administration of the labeled quantity of each dose.

Table Volume of injection

Labelled quantity (ml)	Excess quantity (ml)	
	Mobile liquid	Viscous liquid
0.5	0.10	0.12
1	0.10	0.15
2.	0.15	0.25
5.	0.30	0.50
10	0.50	0.70
20	0.60	0.90
50	1.0	1.5

Procedure Select 5 containers if the labelled quantity is 2 ml or less; 3 containers if the labelled quantity is more than 2 ml to 50 ml. Open the containers with caution to avoid any loss of the contents. Remove individual content of each containers by suitable dry syringes to individual calibrated graduated apparatus, and measure the volume at room temperature. For injections of oily liquids, warm containers and shake thoroughly before removing the volume. The content in each container is not less than the labelled quantity of the injection.

(2) Other tests Other tests, including the test of visible foreign matters, insoluble particles, related substances, and so on, should comply with reguirements stated in tests for injections stipulated by Ch.P.

Huangqi Injection (Huangqi Zhusheye)

It is a preparation recorded in the Pharmaceutics Standards of Health Ministry of People's Republic of China.

The injection is made of radix astragali, which is the dried root of *Astragalus membranaceus* (Fisch.) Bunge. var. *mongholicus* (Bge.) Hsiao or *Astragalus membranaceus* (Fisch.) Bge. (Fam. Leguminosae). The crude drug contains saponin, flavonoid and polysaccharide. The content of astragaloside is not less than 0.08mg/ml in the solution.

Description Yellow, or light brown clear solution.

Action To reinforce qi and strengthen the superficial resistance, and to promote the discharge of pus and the growth of new tissue.

Indications Viral myocarditis and heart function deficiency due to lack of the heart qi, and hepatitis due to deficiency of the spleen with damp pathogen.

Usage and dosage 2 ~ 4ml, im bid . or 10 ~ 20ml, iv, q.d.or ut.dict.

Specification Ampoule 2ml (equal to crud drug 4g), 10ml (equal to crud drug20g).

Storage Protected from light, store sealed.

Exercise materials

Instruments: Flasks (1000ml, 500ml), filter flask Buchner funnel (φ9mm) set with vacuum pump, tubes (10ml), Sintered Glass Filters, water baths, fill/ seal suits, thin layer plates (silica gel G), tanks.

Reagents: Radix Astragali, ethanol, water for injection use, *n* – butanol, chloroform, methanol, astragaloside Ⅳ, and 10% sulfuric acid in ethanol.

Exercise method

1. Prescription

Radix Astragali	2000g
Water for Injection	added up to 1000ml

2. Preparation

(1) Extraction Extract 100 g of Radix Astragali chips for 90 minutes with boiling water three times. Separate and combine the decoction solution. Filter and evaporate filtrate to 50 ml under vacuum.

(2) Refining Precipitate impurities from the concentrate by treating it with 150 ml of

alcohol and refrigerate. Filter and evaporate filtrate to 40 ml under vacuum. Add 230 ml of alcohol to the concentrate, mix and refrigerate. Filter and evaporate filtrate to 10 ml under vacuum. Dilute the fine concentrate with 90 ml of injection water, and refrigerate for 12 h. Filter and evaporate filtrate to 25 ml under vacuum.

(3) Blending Cool the concentrate and adjust pH value to 7.5 with 20% NaOH. Boil the concentrate mixed with 0.125% active charcoal for 5 min, filter before cooling, add injection water up to 50 ml and filter. Adjust pH value of the solution to 7.5 with 20% NaOH and filter with a sintered glass funnel under vacuum.

(4) Filling, sealing and sterilize Fill the solution in 2ml – volume ampoules and seal the ampoules with a fill/seal machine. Sterilize the injection by flowing steam for 30 min.

3. Test and identification

(1) Visible foreign matters of injection is tested according the method regulated officially.

(2) To 1.5ml of the solution add 28 ml of water and extract with 20 ml of water – saturated n – BuOH twice. The combined BuOH extracts are washed twice with 20 ml of water and remove the water phase. The BuOH solution is evaporated to dryness on a water – bath, and the residue is dissolved in 0.5ml of methanol as the test solution. Dissolve 1 mg of astragaloside Ⅳ in 1 ml of methanol to produce a solution as the reference solution. Carry out the method for TLC (Pharmacopoeia of P.R.China, Appendix Ⅳ B) using silica gel G as coating substance and lower layer of chloroform – methanol – water (13:7:2) as the mobile phase. Apply separately to the plate 2 μl of each of the two solutions. After developing and removal of the plate, dry it in air, spray with 10% sulfuric acid in ethanol, and heat at 105℃ until the spots become distinct. A brown spot in the chromatogram obtained with the test solution corresponds in position and colour to the spot in the chromatogram obtained with the reference solution. Examine under UV light (365nm), the same orange – yellow fluorescent spots are shown in both chromatograms.

Questions

1. List the problems of injections made from crude drugs.
2. List the requirements for advantages and disadvantages of parenteral therapy.

Reference

1. Pharmacopoeia Commission of PRC. Pharmacopoeia of P.R.of China. Volume Ⅰ. Beijing: Chemical Industry Press. 2000, 891

2. Health Ministry of P.R.of China. Pharmaceutical Standards of Health Ministry of P.R.of China – Preparations of TCM Vol. 17. Beijing: People's Health PRESS. 1998, 257

实验四　煎　膏　剂

【实验目的】

1．熟悉煎膏剂的制备方法和特点。

2．了解煎膏剂的质量检查。

【实验指导】

煎膏剂[1]系指药材用水煎煮、去渣浓缩后，加炼蜜或糖制成的半流体制剂。

1．制备煎膏剂的一般要求

（1）药材一般需加工成片或段，按具体品种规定的方法煎煮，滤过，滤液浓缩至规定的相对密度，即得清膏。

（2）如果需加入药粉，一般应加入药物细粉。

（3）清膏按规定量加入炼蜜或糖（或转化糖）收膏；若需加药物细粉，待冷却后加入，搅拌混匀。除另有规定外，加炼蜜或糖（转化糖）的量，一般不超过清膏量的3倍。

（4）煎膏剂应无焦臭、异味，无糖的结晶析出。

（5）煎膏剂应密封，置阴凉处贮藏。

2．煎膏剂的检查

（1）相对密度　取供试品适量，精密称定，加水约2倍，精密称定，混匀，作为供试品溶液。照相对密度测定法（参照《中华人民共和国药典》（一部）附录）测定，按下式计算，即得。

$$供试品相对密度=\frac{w_1-w_1\times f}{w_2-w_2\times f}$$

式中　w_1 为比重瓶内供试品溶液的重量，g；

w_2 为比重瓶内水的重量，g；

$$f=\frac{加入供试品中的水重量}{供试品重量+加入供试品中的水重量}$$

凡加药材细粉的煎膏剂，不再检查相对密度，应符合煎膏剂项下的规定。

（2）不溶物　取供试品5g，加热水200ml，搅拌使溶，放置3分钟后观察，不得有焦屑等异物（微量细小纤维、颗粒不在此限）。

加药材细粉的煎膏剂，应在未加入药粉前检查，符合规定后方可加入药粉。加入药粉后不再检查不溶物。

（3）装量　照最低装量检查法（参照《中华人民共和国药典》（一部））检查，应符合规定。

3．辅料的选择与处理：制备煎膏剂的辅料主要有炼蜜和炼糖。

（1）蜂蜜：因生蜜含有水分、杂质等，易霉败，故需炼制。炼制的蜂蜜有三种规格：嫩蜜、中蜜和老蜜。

(2) 炼糖：其目的在于使糖的晶粒熔融，去除水分，净化杂质和杀死微生物。

实验 二 冬 膏

二冬膏（Erdonggao）[2]是《中华人民共和国药典》2000年版一部收载的中药制剂。本品为中药天冬和麦冬制成的煎膏剂。天冬来源于百合科植物天冬 *Asparagus cochinchinensis*（Lour）Merr. 的干燥块根。麦冬来源于百合科植物麦冬 *Ophiopogon japonicus*（Thunb.）Ker-Gawl. 的干燥块根，含多种甾体皂苷。

性状：本品为黄棕色稠厚的半流体；味甜、微苦。

功能与主治：养阴润肺。用于肺阴不足引起的燥咳痰少，痰中带血，鼻干咽痛。

用法与用量：口服，一次9~15g，一日2次。

贮藏：密封，置阴凉处。

【实验材料】

仪器：煎药锅、漏斗（Φ9mm）、纱布、烧杯200ml、500ml、1000ml各1只、普通电炉、玻美比重计、钢筛（200目）、天平等。

药品和试剂：天冬、麦冬、蜂蜜等。

【实验方法】

1. 处方

天冬	500g
麦冬	500g
炼蜜	适量

（学生实验可采用五分之一量）

2. 制法

(1) 煎煮：取以上二味中药共200g，切段后，加入相当于药材12倍量的水，先以武火煮沸后，降低火力，保持微沸，煎煮3次，第一次3小时，第二、三次各2小时，常加以搅拌，然后合并煎液，药渣压榨，压榨液与煎液合并，静置用200目滤器过滤。

(2) 浓缩：将上述滤液直火浓缩成相对密度为1.21~1.25（80℃），或以搅拌棒趁热蘸取浓缩液滴于桑皮纸上，以液滴的周围无渗出水迹时为度，即得清膏。

(3) 收膏：取清膏趁热加炼蜜（每100g清膏加炼蜜50g），混匀。收膏时随着稠度的增加，加热温度可相应降低，并需不断搅拌和掠去液面上的浮沫。收膏稠度为相对密度1.4（80℃）左右。

(4) 分装：将上述煎膏充分放冷后再装入适宜的容器中，然后加盖，切勿在热时加盖，以免水蒸气冷凝回入煎膏中，久贮后易产生霉败现象。

3. 鉴别和检查

应符合煎膏剂项下有关的各项规定。

实验　益母草膏

益母草膏（Yimucao gao）[3]是《中华人民共和国药典》2000年版一部收载的中药制剂。本品为中药益母草制成的煎膏剂。益母草来源于唇形科植物益母草 *Leonurus japonicus* Sweet. 的新鲜或干燥地上部分，含益母草碱、水苏碱等多种生物碱。

性状：本品为棕黑色稠厚的半流体；气微，味苦、甜。

功能与主治：活血调经。用于经闭，痛经及产后淤血腹痛。

用法与用量：口服，一次10g，一日1～2次。

注意：孕妇禁用。

贮藏：密封，置阴凉处。

【实验材料】

仪器：煎药锅、漏斗（Φ9mm）、纱布、烧杯（200ml、500ml、1000ml各1只）、普通电炉、玻美比重计、200目钢筛、层析展开缸、喷雾瓶、天平、显微镜等。

药品和试剂：益母草、红糖等。

【实验方法】

1．处方

益母草	100g
红糖	适量

2．制法

（1）煎煮：取上述益母草，切碎后，加入相当于药材10倍量的水，先以武火煮沸后，降低火力，保持微沸，煎煮2次，每次2小时，常加以搅拌，然后合并煎液，药渣压榨，压榨液与煎液合并，静置，用200目滤器过滤。

（2）浓缩：将上述滤液直火浓缩成相对密度为1.21～1.25（80℃），或以搅拌棒趁热蘸取浓缩液滴于桑皮纸上，以液滴的周围无渗出水迹时为度。即得清膏。

（3）收膏：取清膏趁热加入红糖（每100g清膏加红糖200g），加热溶化，混匀。收膏时，随着稠度的增加，加热温度可相应降低，并需不断搅拌和掠去液面上的浮沫。收膏稠度为相对密度1.4（80℃）左右。

（4）分装：将上述煎膏充分放冷后再装入适宜的容器中，然后加盖，切勿在热时加盖，以免水蒸气冷凝回入煎膏中，久贮后易产生霉败现象。

3．检查

（1）10g益母草膏溶于20ml水中，该溶液的相对密度应为1.10～1.12（参见《中华人民共和国药典》附录）。

（2）应符合煎膏剂的有关要求。

【思考题】

1．制备炼蜜、炼糖的目的和要求是什么？

2．简述煎膏剂返砂的原因及处理办法。

参 考 文 献

1．国家药典委员会．中华人民共和国药典（一部）．北京：化学工业出版社．2000，附录
2．国家药典委员会．中华人民共和国药典（一部）．北京：化学工业出版社．2000，324
3．国家药典委员会．中华人民共和国药典（一部）．北京：化学工业出版社．2000，566

Exercise 4 Concentrated Decoctions

Learning objectives

1. Practice and learn the general process to produce concentrated decoctions.
2. Understand the characteristics and the quality control of concentrated decoctions.

Instruction

Concentrated decoctions[1] are semi – fluid preparations prepared by decocting the crude drugs in water, concentrating after discarding the residue and adding honey or sugar.

1. General requirement for preparation of the production and storage of concentrated decoctions

(1) The crude drugs should be processed to slices or sections, decocted according to the appropriate methods for specific species and filtered. The extract is obtained by concentrating the filtrate to a specified relative density.

(2) The fine powder of drugs should be added when the powder is needed as required.

(3) The extract is concentrated by adding specified quantity of processed honey or sugar (or invert sugar). The fine powder of crude drugs should be added into a cold concentrated decoction, stirred and mixed well. The quantity of honey or sugar (or invert sugar) added is generally not more than 3 times of that of the extract, unless otherwise specified.

(4) Concentrated decoctions should have no burnt or other abnormal odour, and have no sugar crystallizes out.

(5) Concentrated decoctions should be preserved in tightly closed containers, stored in a cool place.

2. Tests

(1) Relative density Weigh accurately a sufficient quantity of concentrated decoction being examined, dilute with 2 quantities of water, weigh accurately and mix well. To determinate the relative density (Ch.P. Appendix), calculate as the following formula.

$$\text{Relative density of concentrated decoction} = \frac{w_1 - w_1 \times f}{w_2 - w_2 \times f}$$

Where w_1 is the weight (g) of concentrated decoction in pycnometer;

w_2 is the weight (g) of water in pycnometer.

$$f = \frac{\text{weight of water added in concentrated decoction}}{\text{weight of concentrated decoction} + \text{weight of water added in concentrated decoction}}$$

It is not necessary to examine the relative density when concentrated decoctions contain fine powder of crude drugs. It should comply with the requirements of specified concentrated decoctions.

(2) Insoluble materials To 5g of the concentrated decoction add 200 ml of hot water, stir to dissolve, allow to stand for 3 minutes, and observe. No foreign matters such as scorched masses, etc. should be observed (a small amount of fine fibres and particles are not defined in this limit).

The concentrated decoction containing fine powder of crude drugs should be examined before the powder is added. The powder is added if it complies with the requirements. It is not necessary to examine the insoluble materials after the powder is added.

(3) Packing weight Carry out the test as described under the lowest packing weight test (Ch.P.Appendix), it should comply with the specified requirement.

3. Selection and processes of excipients: The main excipients are process (refined) honey and process (refined) sugar.

(1) Honey: Since crude honey is perishable, containing water, impurities, etc., refinement of the crude honey is necessary. The refined honey is classified into: tender honey, middle honey and tough honey.

(2) Sugar: Processes of sugar is to melt sugar crystals, evaporate water, destroy impurities and kill microorganism.

Erdong Gao

Erdong Concentrated Decoction[2] is a preparation recorded in the Pharmacopoeia of People's Republic of China. The decoction is made of Radix Asparagi, original from *Asparagus cochinchinensis* (Lour) Merr, and Radix Ophiopogonis original from *Ophiopogon japonicus* (Thunb.) Ker – Gawl, containing many kinds of steroid glycosides.

Description A brownish – yellow viscous semifluid; taste, sweet and slightly bitter.

Action To nourish yin of the lung.

Indications Dry cough with scanty expectoration, bloody sputum, dry nose and sore throat.

Usage and dosage 9 ~ 15g, 2 times a day.

Storage Preserve in tightly closed containers, stored in shade and cool place.

Exercise materials

Instruments: decocting pan, funnel, gauze, beakers, hotplate, hydrometer, screens, scale, etc.

Drugs and reagents: Radix Asparagi, Radix Ophiopogonis, and honey, etc.

Exercise method

1. Formulation

Radix Asparagi	100g;
Radix Ophiopogonis	100g.
Honey	*q.s.*

2. Procedure

(1) Decoction　Decoct the two ingredients with 2400 ml of water three times (3, 2 and 2 hours respectively). Combine the decoctions, stand, filter with a sieve (200 mesh).

(2) Concentration　Evaporate the filtrate to an extract with relative density of 1.21 ~ 1.25 (80 ~ 85℃), or indicated with a piece of paper made of mulberry bark: drop the concentrate on the paper, if there is no water spreading on the paper it is right.

(3) Collection　To each 100 g of the extract add 50g of refined honey and mix well, cool down with stirring and clear foam on the face. The relative density of the collected decoction is about 1.4 (80℃).

(4) Package　The collected decoction should be cool exactly, and then put in a suitable container closed with a lid. Otherwise, as the decoction cool from a hot state, it may become moldy if steam drops back in the decoction.

3. Tests

Complies with the general requirements for concentrated decoctions.

Extractum Leonuri Inspissatum

Concentrated Decoction of Motherwort Herb[3] is the concentrated decoction prepared from Herba Leonuri original from the fresh or dry aerial part of *Leonurus japonicus* Sweet. The medication is recorded in the Pharmacopoeia of People's Republic of China.

Description　A brownish-black and thick semifluid; odour, slight; taste, bitter and sweet.

Action　To activate blood circulation and regulate menstruation.

Indications　Amenorrhea, dysmenorrhea, abdominal pain after parturition due to blood stasis.

Usage and dosage　10g, 1 ~ 2 times a day.

Precaution　Contraindicated in pregnancy.

Storage　Preserve in tightly closed containers, stored in a shade and cool place.

Exercise materials

Instruments: decocting pan, funnel, gauze, beakers, hotplate, hydrometer, screens, scale, etc.

Drugs and reagents: Herba Leonuri, brown sugar, etc.

Exercise Method

1. Formulation

Herba Leonuri	100g
Brown sugar	*q.s.*

2. Procedure

(1) Decoction Cut Herba Leonuri, decoct with 1000 ml of water for two times, often stir, 2 hours each, combine the decoctions, stand, filter with a sieve (200 mesh).

(2) Concentration Concentrate the filtrate to a clear concentrated decoction of relative density 1.21 ~ 1.25 (deternlined at 80 ~ 85℃), or indicated with a piece of paper made of mulberry bark: drop the concentrate on the paper, if there is no water spreading on the paper it is right.

(3) Collection To each 100 g of clear concentrated decoction add 200 g of brown sugar, heat to dissolve, mix well. Lower the temperature with stirring and clear foam on the face. The collected last concentrate is at the specified relative density of 1.4 (80℃) or so.

(4) Package: The collected decoction should be cooled exactly, and then put in a suitable container closed with a lid. Otherwise when the decoction cool from a hot state, it could become moldy if steam drops back in the decoction.

3. Tests

(1) Relative density 1.10 ~ 1.12, in a solution of 10 g in 20 ml of water (Ch.P.Appendix).

(2) Complies with the general requirements for concentrated decoctions.

Questions

1. What are purposes and requirements of process honey and process sugar?

2. Describe the cause of sugar crystallization on the concentrated decoction. What are the methods for solving the problem?

References

1. Pharmacopoeia Commission of PRC. Pharmacopoeia of the People's Republic of China Volume I. Beijing: Chemical Industry Press. 2000, Appendix

2. Pharmacopoeia Commission of PRC. Pharmacopoeia of the People's Republic of China (English edition). Volume I. Beijing: Chemical Industry Press. 1997, 268

3. Pharmacopoeia Commission of PRC. Pharmacopoeia of the People's Republic of China (English edition). Volume I. Beijing: Chemical Industry Press. 1997, 275, 324

实验五　软　膏　剂

【实验目的】

1．熟悉中药软膏剂的质量要求。

2．通过紫草膏和老鹳草膏的制备，掌握中药软膏剂的一般制法。

【实验指导】

软膏剂[1]系指药物、药材、药材提取物与适宜基质制成具有适当稠度的膏状外用制剂。常用基质分为油脂性、水溶性和乳剂型基质。其中用乳剂型基质制成的软膏剂亦称乳膏剂。

1．制备中药软膏剂的一般要求

软膏剂在生产与贮藏期间均应符合下列有关规定：

(1) 膏剂常用的基质材料有凡士林、液状石蜡、羊毛脂 、蜂蜡 、植物油、单硬脂酸甘油酯、高级脂肪醇、聚乙二醇、淀粉甘油、甘油明胶、羧甲基纤维素钠和乳化剂等。

(2) 供制软膏剂用的固体药物，除在某一组分中溶解或共熔者外，应预先用适宜的方法制成细粉。

(3) 软膏剂应均匀、细腻、具有适当的黏稠性，易涂布在皮肤或黏膜上并无刺激性；必要时可加入透皮吸收促进剂和表面活性剂。

(4) 软膏剂应无酸败、异臭、变色、变硬、油水分离等变质现象，必要时可加适量防腐剂或抗氧剂。

(5) 软膏剂所用的包装材料不得与药物或基质发生理化反应。

(6) 除另有规定外，软膏剂应置遮光容器中密闭贮存。

2．软膏剂的检查

(1) 微生物　按照微生物限度检查法或无菌检查法检查（参见《中华人民共和国药典》附录）应符合规定。

(2) 装量检查　按照最低装量检查法检查（参见《中华人民共和国药典》附录），应符合规定。

(3) 粒度　含药材细粉的软膏剂检查粒度（参见《中华人民共和国药典》附录）。

实验　紫　草　膏

紫草膏[2]（zicao gao）是《中华人民共和国药典（一部）》收载的中药制剂。本品为紫草等中药制成的软膏。紫草来源于紫草科植物新疆紫草 *Arnebia euchroma*（Royle）Johnst.，紫草 *Lithospermum erythrorhizon* Sieb. et Zucc. 或内蒙紫草 *Arnebia guttata* Bunge 的干燥根。新疆紫草和紫草含紫草素等醌类成分。此外，本品含有大量挥发性有效成分。

性状：本品为紫红色的软膏；具特殊的油腻气。

功能与主治：化腐生肌。用于疮疡，痈疽已溃。

用法与用量：外用，摊于纱布上贴患处，每隔1~2日换药一次。

贮藏：密封，置阴凉干燥处。

【实验材料】

仪器：烧瓶（500ml）、布氏漏斗（Φ9mm）、烧杯（50ml，200ml）、冷凝管、水浴、普通天平、刮刀、药勺等。

药品和试剂：紫草、当归、防风、地黄、白芷、乳香、没药、食用植物油、蜂蜡等。

【实验方法】

1．处方

紫草	500g
当归	150g
防风	150g
地黄	150g
白芷	150g
乳香	150g
没药	150g
植物油	6000g
蜂蜡	适量

（学生可以用百分之一量实验）

2．制法

（1）粉碎：乳香、没药粉碎成细粉，过筛。

（2）提取：当归、防风、地黄、白芷等四味药酌予碎断，另取食用植物油60g，同置锅内炸枯，去渣；将紫草用水湿润，置锅内炸至油呈紫红色，去渣，滤过。

（3）制软膏：取蜂蜡适量加入上述油溶液（每10g植物油加蜂蜡2~4g）熔化，待温，加入上述粉末，搅匀，即得。

3．检查

应符合软膏剂有关的各项规定。

实验　老鹳草软膏

老鹳草软膏[3]（Laoguancao Ruangao）是《中华人民共和国药典（一部）》收载的中药制剂。本品为中药老鹳草制成的软膏。老鹳草来源于牛儿苗 *Erodium stephanianum* Willd. 或老鹳草 *Geranium Wilfordii* Maxim. 的干燥地上部分。老鹳草含大量鞣质类化合物。

性状：本品为褐紫色的软膏。

功能与主治：除湿解毒，收敛生肌。用于湿毒蕴结所致的湿疹，痈、疔、疮、疖及小面积水、火烫伤。

用法与用量：外用，涂敷患处，一日1次。

贮藏：密闭。

【实验材料】

仪器：烧瓶（500ml）、布氏漏斗（Φ9mm）、烧杯（50ml，200ml）、冷凝管、水浴、普通天平、刮刀、药勺等。

药品和试剂：老鹳草、乙醇、羊毛脂、凡士林、对羟基苯甲酸乙酯等。

【实验方法】

1．处方

老鹳草	1000g
羊毛脂	50g
对羟基苯甲酸乙酯	0.3g
凡士林	适量
制成软膏	1000g

（学生实验可用二十分之一量）

2．制法

（1）提取：取老鹳草50g，加300ml水适量煎煮二次，每次1小时，合并煎液，滤过，滤液浓缩至50～60ml。加等量乙醇使沉淀，静置12～24小时，滤取上清液，浓缩成稠膏。

（2）制软膏：取相当于药材50g的老鹳草稠膏，加羟苯乙酯0.015g、羊毛脂2.5g与凡士林至50g，混匀，即得。

3．鉴别

取本品5g，加乙醇10ml，置水浴上搅拌使溶化，放冷，滤过，除去凝固的凡士林，取滤液1ml，加三氯化铁试液1～2滴，即显深蓝色，放置后变蓝黑色；另取滤液2ml，加0.25%硫酸铜溶液，即生成白色沉淀；再取滤液2ml，加氯化钙试液，即生成白色沉淀。

4．检查

应符合软膏剂的有关规定。

实验　乳剂型软膏基质

乳剂基质是一种黏性液体或半固体，分为油/水型和水/油型。油/水型的基质可用于剃须、护手以及做为其他乳膏的基质。水/油型的基质可用于冷霜、润肤剂以及做为其他乳膏的基质。这两种基质具有不同的物理特性。在基质中加入合适的药物可用于皮肤和黏膜疾病的外部治疗。现选择一种油/水型的基质作为练习。

【实验材料】

仪器：蒸发皿、水浴、小烧杯。

试剂：见处方。

【实验方法】

1．处方

硬脂酸		2.4g
单硬脂酸甘油酯		0.7g
液体石蜡		1.2g
白凡士林		0.2g
羊毛脂		1.0g
三乙醇胺		0.08g
蒸馏水	加至	20.0g

2．制法

将硬脂酸、单硬脂酸甘油酯、液体石蜡、白凡士林、和羊毛脂放入蒸发皿中，在水浴上加热至80℃左右溶解。将三乙醇胺和适量蒸馏水放入蒸发皿中，同样在浴上加热至80℃左右溶解。在两种混合物都达到合适的时候，在水浴上混合、连续搅拌几分钟，然后在室温下搅拌至冷凝。

3．检查

(1) 外观。

(2) 油/水型乳剂的物理特性（参见《中药药剂学》教科书）。

【思考题】

1．制备软膏剂的基本要求是什么？

2．软膏剂常用基质可分为三类，老鹳草软膏使用的是哪种基质？为什么？

3．评价紫草膏的制备方法，并设计一种新的制备工艺。

3．试设计一种乳剂性软膏基质。

4．油/水型和水/油型乳剂在物理性质上有何不同？

参 考 文 献

1．中华人民共和国药典委员会．《中华人民共和国药典（一部）》北京：化学工业出版社．2000，附录14

2．中华人民共和国药典委员会．《中华人民共和国药典（一部）》北京：化学工业出版社．2000，280，600

3．中华人民共和国药典委员会．《中华人民共和国药典（一部）》北京：化学工业出版社．2000，91，443

Exercise 5 Ointment

Exercise objectives

1. Practice and learn the general process to produce ointments made from Chinese herbs.

2. Understand the quality control of the ointment.

Introduction

Ointments[1] are paste – like preparations with a suitable consistency, usually containing medicaments, crude drugs and their extracts incorporated in a suitable base, and intended for external application to the skin. The bases mainly used in preparation of Ointments may be classified into fatty bases, water – soluble bases and emulsifying bases. Ointments with emulsion bases are usually known as creams.

1. General requirements of the production of Ointments

The production and storage of the ointments should comply with the following requirements.

(1) Vaseline, liquid paraffin, lanolin, beeswax, vegetable oils, glycerin monostearate, stearyl alcohol, polyethylene glycols, starch – glycerin, glycerinated gelatin, sodium carboxymethyl cellulose and suitable emulsifying agents may be used as bases in the preparation of ointments.

(2) In the preparation of ointments, solid medicaments should be powdered finely before use in addition to their dissolution in or formation of a eutectic mixture with one of the ingredients.

(3) Ointments should be uniform and emollient to apply to the skin with no irritating action but with proper consistency. Skin penetration enhancers and surfactants may be added if necessary.

(4) Ointments should show no evidence of deterioration such as rancidity, foreign odour, discoloration, hardening, or a separation of oil and water. Preservatives or antioxidants may be added to the ointments.

(5) Containers for ointments should not interact physically or chemically with the medicaments or bases.

(6) Unless otherwise stated, ointments should be preserved in well – closed containers, protected from light.

2. Tests

(1) Microbiological test Comply with the requirements stated under microbial limit test (See Ch.P.Appendix).

(2) Comply with the test for minimum fill (See Ch.P.Appendix).

(3) Granularity Granulometry should be conducted for the ointement containing crude drug powders (See Ch.P. Appendix).

Zicao Ointment

Zicao ointment[2] is a preparation Chinese Traditional Medica recorded in the Pharmacopoeia of the people's Republic of China. The ointment is made from Chinese traditional herbs zicao, etc. Zicao originates from the dried root of *Arnebia euchroma* (Royle) Johnst., or *Lithospermum erythrorhizon* Sieb. et Zucc., or *Arnebia guttata* Bunge. Radix Arnebiae and Radix Lithospermi contain quinones such as shikonin, etc.

Description: A purplish – red ointment, with a characteristic oily odour.

Action: To heal the dead tissue and promote the growth of the new tissue.

Indications: Boil or abscess that has bursted.

Usage and Dosage: Spread on a piece of gauze for topical application. Change the dressing every 1 ~ 2 days.

Storage: Preserve in tightly closed containers, stored in a cool and dry place.

Exercise materials

Instruments: flask (500ml), beaker (50ml, 200ml), Buchner funnel (Φ9mm), condenser, water bath, balance, scraper, and so on.

Drugs and reagents: Radix Arnebiae or Radix Lithospermi, Radix Angelicae Sinensis, Radix saposhnikoviae, Radix Rehmanniae, Radix Angelicae Dahuricae, Olibanum, Myrrh, edible vegetable oil, beeswax and so on.

Exercise method

1. Formulation

Radix Arnebiae and Radix Lithospermi	500g
Radix Angelicae Sinensis	150g
Radix Saposhnikoviae	150g
Radix Rehmanniae	150g
Radix Angelicae Dahuricae	150g
Olibanum	150g
Myrrh	150g

vegetable oil 6000g

beeswax q.s.

(One percent of the quantity may be used for a student's exercise.)

2. Procedure

(1) Pulverize olibanum and myrrh to fine powders, sift. Cut radix angelicae sinensis, radix saposhnikoviae, radix rehmanniae, and radix angelicae dahuricae properly, then fry with 60g of edible vegetable oil, and discard the residue. Soften radix Arnebiae or radix Lithospermi with water, deep - dry until the oil becomes purplish - red in colour, discard the residue, filter.

(2) Add a appropriate quantity of beeswax (to each 10g of oil add 2 ~ 4g of beeswax), melt, and stir well the above powders while hot.

3. Tests

Comply with the general requirements for ointments.

Unguentum Geranii (Common Heron's Bill Ointment)

Common heron's bill ointment[3] is a preparation Chinese Traditional Medica recorded in Pharmacopoeia of the people's Republic of China. The Ointment is made from the dried aerial part of *Erodium stephanianum* Willd. (Common Heron's Bill Herb) or *Geranium wilfordii* Maxim. It contains many tannin compounds.

Description A brownish - purple ointment.

Action To counteract inflammation, to arrest discharges, and to promote the growth of the new tissue.

Indication Eczema, carbuncles, boils, or sores, and scalds and burns of small area.

Usage and Dosage To be applied topically, once a day.

Storage Preserve in well closed containers.

Exercise materials

Instruments: flask (500ml), beaker (50ml, 200ml), Buchner funnel (Φ9mm), condenser tube, water bath, balance, scraper blade, etc.

Drugs and reagents: Herba Erodii seu Geranii, ethanol, wool fat, vaseline, ethyl *p* - hydroxybenzoate, etc.

Exercise method

1. Formulation

Herba Erodii seu Geranii 1000g

Wool fat	50g
Ethyl *p* – hydroxybenzoate	0.3g
Vaseline	q.s.

Make up to 1000g.

2. Procedure

(1) Extraction Decoct 50g of Herba Erodii seu Gerantii with 300ml water twice, for 1 hour each time. Combine the decoctions, filter, concentrate the filtrate to 50 ~ 60ml, and add the same amount of ethanol to precipitate. Allow to stand for 12 ~ 24 hours, filter the supernatant and concentrate.

(2) Making ointment Add ethyl *p* – hydroxybenzoate 0.015g, wool fat 2.5g and vaseline to the extract (the total weight is about 1000g), mix thoroughly and the ointment is completed.

3. Identification

Dissolve by stirring 5g in 10ml of ethanol on a water bath, cool and filter to remove the solidified vaseline. To 1ml of the filtrate, add 1 to 2 drops of ferric chloride TS, a dark blue colour is produced, which turns to bluish – black after standing. To another 2ml of the filtrate add 0.25% cupric sulfate solution, a white precipitate is produced. To another 2ml of the filtrate add calcium chloride solution, a white precipitate is produced.

4. Tests

Comply with the general requirements for ointments.

Emulsion base of Ointment

Emulsion bases are viscous liquid or semisolid emulsions of either the oil/water (O/W) or water/oil (W/O) type. O/W type bases may be used for shaving, hand, and foundation creams and W/O type bases for cold and emollient creams, and other ointments. The two types of bases have different physical properties. The bases contain medicinal substances are intended for the external application to the skin or mucous membranes. This exercise is to prepare an oil/water type bases.

Exercise materials

Instruments: Porcelain evaporating dish, water – bath, and small beaker.

Reagents: See the formulation.

Exercise method

1. Formulation

Stearic acid	2.4g

Glycerin monostearate		0.7g
Liquid paraffin		1.2g
White petrolatum		0.2g
Lanolin		1.0g
Triethanolamine		0.08g
Distilled water	q.s. to	20.0g

2. Procedure

Dissolve stearic acid, glycerin monostearate, liquid paraffin, white petrolatum, and lanolin together using a steam bath till at the temperature of 80℃ remove from heat. Dissolve triethanolamine in water using a steam bath till at the temperature of 80℃. After both mixtures are at appropriate temperatures add them together stirring rapidly for several minutes and stirring continuously at room temperature until it has congealed.

3. Test

(1) Appearance.

(2) Physical properties (See《Pharmaceutics of TCM》used for the lecture course.)

Question

1. Describe the common requirements of the production of the ointments.
2. Which kind of bases did the Common Heron's Bill Ointment use? What is the reason for the choice?
3. Evaluate the preparation method of zicao ointment, and design a new method to produce the medication.
4. Try to design a cream matrix.
5. What differences are there between oil/water (O/W) and water/oil (W/O) type emulsions in physical properties?

Reference

1. Pharmacopoeia Commission of PRC. Pharmacopoeia of the People's Republic of China (English Edition). Volume Ⅰ, Beijing: Chemical Industry Press, 1997, Appendix A-11
2. Pharmacopoeia Commission of PRC. Pharmacopoeia of the People's Republic of China Volume Ⅰ, Beijing: Chemical Industry Press, 2000. 280, 600
3. Pharmacopoeia Commission of PRC. Pharmacopoeia of the People's Republic of China Volume Ⅰ, Beijing: Chemical Industry Press, 2000, 91, 443

实验六　丸　　剂

【实验目的】

1. 了解丸剂的制备方法及特点。
2. 掌握塑制法制备蜜丸。
3. 了解丸剂的质量检查。

【实验指导】

丸剂[1]系指药材细粉或药材提取物加适宜的黏合剂或其他辅料制成的球形或类球形固体制剂，分为蜜丸、水蜜丸、水丸、糊丸、浓缩丸、蜡丸和微丸等类型。

蜜丸系指药材细粉以蜂蜜为黏合剂制成的丸剂。水蜜丸系指药材细粉以蜂蜜和水为黏合剂制成的丸剂。水丸系指药材细粉以水（或根据制法用黄酒、醋、稀药汁、糖液等）黏合制成的丸剂。糊丸系指药材细粉以米糊或面糊等为黏合剂制成的丸剂。浓缩丸系指药材或部分药材提取的清膏或浸膏，与适宜的辅料或药物细粉，以水、蜂蜜或蜂蜜和水为黏合剂制成的丸剂。根据所用黏合剂的不同，分为浓缩水丸、浓缩蜜丸和浓缩水蜜丸。蜡丸系指药材细粉以蜂蜡为黏合剂制成的丸剂。微丸系指直径小于2.5mm的各类丸剂。

根据生产方法的不同，丸剂又可分为三类，即塑制丸、泛制丸和滴制丸，三类丸剂使用的丸材也不相同，作用特点也不同。

1. 制备和贮藏丸剂的一般要求

(1) 除另有规定外，供制丸剂用的药粉应为细粉或最细粉（能通过5号筛或6号筛）。

(2) 用蜂蜜须经炼制后使用。按炼蜜程度分为嫩蜜、中蜜和老蜜，制备蜜丸时可根据品种、气候等具体情况选用。除另有规定外，用搓丸法制备蜜丸时，炼蜜应趁热加入药粉中，混合均匀；处方中有树脂类、胶类及含挥发性成分的药物时，炼蜜应在60℃左右加入；用泛丸法制备水蜜丸时，炼蜜应用开水稀释后使用。

(3) 丸所用清膏或浸膏应按制法规定，采用煎煮、渗漉等方法取煎液、漉液浓缩制成。

(4) 除另有规定外水蜜丸、水丸、浓缩水蜜丸和浓缩水丸均应在80℃以下进行干燥。含挥发性成分或淀粉较多的丸剂（包括糊丸）应在60℃以下进行干燥；不宜加热干燥的应采用其他适宜的方法进行干燥。

(5) 蜡丸所用的蜂蜡应符合药典该药材项下规定。使用前应除去蜂蜡中的杂质。制备蜡丸时，将蜂蜡加热熔化，待冷却至60℃左右按比例加入药粉，混合均匀，趁热按蜜丸制法制丸，并注意保温。

(6) 凡需包衣和打光的丸剂，应使用各该品种制法规定的包衣材料进行包衣和打光。

(7) 丸剂外观应圆整均匀，色泽一致。大蜜丸和小蜜丸应细腻滋润、软硬适中。蜡丸表面应光滑无裂纹，丸内不得有蜡点和颗粒。

(8) 丸剂应密封贮藏。蜡丸应密封并置阴凉干燥处贮藏。

2．丸剂的检查

（1）水分　照水分测定法（参照《中华人民共和国药典》（一部）附录Ⅸ H）测定。除另有规定外，大蜜丸、小蜜丸、浓缩蜜丸中所含水分不得过15.0%；水蜜丸、浓缩水蜜丸不得过12.0%；水丸、糊丸和浓缩水丸不得过9.0%；微丸按其所属丸剂类型的规定判定。蜡丸不检查水分。

（2）重量差异　按丸服用的丸剂照第一法检查，按重量服用的丸剂照第二法检查。

第一法　一般以一次服用量最高丸数为1份（详见《中国药典》附录），供试品10份，分别称定重量，再与标示总量（一次服用最高丸数×每丸标示量）或标示重量相比较，应符合表1的规定。超出重量差异限度的不得多于2份，并不得有1份超出限度一倍。

第二法　取供试品10丸为1份，供取10份，分别称定重量，求得平均值，每份重量与平均值相比较（有标示量的与标示量相比较），应符合表2的规定。超出重量差异限度的不得多于2份，并不得有1份超出限度一倍。

包糖衣的丸剂应在包衣前检查丸芯的重量差异，符合表2规定后，方可包糖衣。包糖衣后不再检查重量差异。

（3）装量差异　单剂量分装的丸剂，装量差异限度应符合表3规定。

检查法　取供试品10袋（瓶），分别称定每袋（瓶）内容物的重量，每袋（瓶）重量与标示装量相比较，应符合表3的规定。超出重量差异限度的不得多于2袋（瓶），并不得有1袋（瓶）超出限度一倍。

（4）溶散时限　除另有规定外，取供试品6丸，选择适当孔径筛网的吊篮（丸剂直径在2.5mm以下的用孔径约0.42mm的筛网，在2.5～3.5mm之间的用孔径1.0mm的筛网，在3.5mm以上的用孔径约2.0mm的筛网），照崩解时限检查法片剂项下的方法（参照《中华人民共和国药典》（一部）附录）加档板进行检查，除另有规定外，小蜜丸、水蜜丸和水丸应在1小时内全部溶散；浓缩丸和糊丸应在2小时内全部溶散；微丸的溶散时限按所属丸剂类型的规定判定，如操作过程中供试品黏附档板妨碍检查时，应另取供试品6丸，不加档板进行检查。

上述检查应在规定时间内全部通过筛网。如有细小颗粒状物未通过筛网，但已软化无硬心者可作合格论。

蜡丸照崩解时限检查法，参照《中华人民共和国药典》有关检查法检查，应符合规定。

大蜜丸不检查溶散时限。

表1.

标示总量	重量差异限度
0.05g或0.05g以下	±12%
0.05g以上至0.1g	±11%
0.1g以上至0.3g	±10%
0.3g以上至1.5g	±9%
1.5g以上至3g	±8%
3g以上至6g	±7%
6g以上至9g	±6%
9g以上	±5%

表 2.

每份的平均重量	重量差异限度
0.05g 或 0.05g 以下	± 12%
0.05g 以上至 0.1g	± 11%
0.1g 以上至 0.3g	± 10%
0.3g 以上至 1g	± 8%
1g 以上至 2g	± 7%
2g 以上	± 6%

表 3.

标示装量	装量差异限度
0.5g 或 0.5g 以下	± 12%
0.5g 以上至 1g	± 11%
1g 以上至 2g	± 10%
2g 以上至 3g	± 8%
3g 以上至 6g	± 6%
6g 以上至 9g	± 5%
9g 以上	± 4%

实验　麻仁润肠丸

麻仁润肠丸（Marenrunchangwan）为《中华人民共和国药典》收载的中药制剂[2]。本品为中药火麻仁、苦杏仁、大黄、木香、陈皮、白芍等制成的大蜜丸。火麻仁来源于大麻（*Cannabis sativa* L.）。其果仁含大量的脂肪油；苦杏仁为杏（*Prunus armeniaca* L.）或山杏（*P. armeniaca* L. Var. Ansu Maxim.）的种子，质润多油；大黄为掌叶大黄（*Rheum palmatum* L.）、唐古特大黄（*Rheum tanguticum* Ma－xim. ex Balf.）或药用大黄（*Rheum officinale* Baill.）的干燥根及根茎，其中的致泻成分为番泻苷。

性状：本品为黄褐色的大蜜丸；气微香，味苦、微甘。

功能与主治：润肠通便。用于肠胃积热。胸腹胀满，大便秘结。

用法与用量：口服，一次 1～2 丸，一日 2 次。

注意：孕妇忌服。

规格：每丸重 6g。

贮藏：密封。

【实验材料】

仪器：普通电炉、天平、钢筛、制丸机、捏合机、崩解仪等。

药品和试剂：火麻仁、苦杏仁、大黄、木香、陈皮、白芍等。

【实验方法】

1. 处方

火麻仁	120g
苦杏仁（去皮炒）	60g
大黄	120g
木香	60g
陈皮	120g
白芍	60g
炼蜜	适量

2. 制法

(1) 药材处理：将上述六味药材粉碎成细粉，过五号钢筛，混匀即可。

(2) 制丸块：将上述已混合均匀的药材细粉按每100g粉末加140～160g炼蜜（老蜜），置于捏合机中充分混匀，使成软硬适宜，可塑性较大的丸块。以能随意塑形而不开裂，手搓捏而不粘手为宜。

(3) 成丸、干燥：将已混匀的丸块放入制丸机中，制成蜜丸。

3. 检查

应符合丸剂检查项下有关的各项规定。

实验　二　至　丸

二至丸（Erzhiwan）是《中华人民共和国药典》收载的中药制剂[3]。本品为中药女贞子、墨旱莲制成的丸剂。女贞子来源于木犀草科植物女贞（*Ligustrum lucidum* Ait.）的干燥成熟果实。墨旱莲来源于菊科植物鳢肠（*Eclipta prostrata* L.）的干燥地上部分。本品为部分药材提取的浸膏，与药物细粉，以蜂蜜和水为黏合剂制成的丸剂。女贞子的主要有效成分为齐墩果酸和多糖。

性状：本品为黑褐色的水蜜丸；气微，味甘而苦。

功能与主治：补益肝肾，滋阴止血。用于肝肾阴虚，眩晕耳鸣，咽干鼻燥，腰膝酸痛，月经量多。

用法与用量：口服，一次9g，一日2次。

贮藏：密封。

【实验材料】

仪器：漏斗（Φ9mm）、纱布、烧杯（200ml、500ml、1000ml各1只）、煎药锅、普通电炉、天平、钢筛、泛丸埚、崩解仪等。

药品和试剂：女贞子、墨旱莲、蜂蜜等。

【实验方法】

1．处方

女贞子	500g
墨旱莲	500g
炼蜜	60g
水	适量

（学生实验取五分之一量）

2．制法

（1）药材处理：将上述女贞子药材粉碎成过六号筛的细粉。取墨旱莲加水600ml煎煮1小时，共两次，合并煎液，药渣压榨，压榨液与煎液合并，滤过，滤液浓缩至相对密度为1.2～1.3（80℃）左右，加炼蜜12g及水适量，混匀，制成黏合剂。

（2）泛制成丸：取3g女贞子细粉，加适量水制成松散的软材，压过二号筛，制成小颗粒，在泛丸锅中滚动，形成模子，筛分后，置于泛丸锅中，喷入上述黏合剂，加入剩余女贞子细粉，泛制成丸。泛丸时，各组学生合并操作。

（3）塑制成丸：将女贞子细粉和黏合剂，充分和匀，制成可塑性丸块，用制丸板制成丸条、丸粒，搓圆。

3．干燥： 将成丸在70～80℃下干燥。

4．检查

(1) 除溶散时限检查应在2小时内溶散外，其他应符合丸剂检查项下的有关的各项规定。

【思考题】

通过实验，你对塑制法和泛制法制丸的特点有何体会和经验？何种方法制备二至丸较好？

参 考 文 献

1．中华人民共和国药典委员会．中华人民共和国药典（一部）．北京：化学工业出版社．2000，附录5．
2．中华人民共和国药典委员会．中华人民共和国药典（一部）．北京：化学工业出版社．2000，584．
3．中华人民共和国药典委员会．中华人民共和国药典（一部）．北京：化学工业出版社．2000，324．

Exercise 6 Pills

Learning objectives

1. Learn the general process to produce pills made from natural medicinal materials.
2. Practice and learn preparation of honeyed pills by kneading and rubbing method.
3. Understand the quality control of the pills.

Instruction

Pills[1] are spherical solid dosage forms made of fine powdered drugs or crude drug extracts, proper binders or other excipients. They are classified into honeyed pills, water-honeyed pills, watered pills, pasted pills, concentrated pills and micro-pills.

Honeyed pills are made of fine powder of crude drugs, using honey as binder. Water-honeyed pills are made of fine powder of crude drugs, using honey and water as binders.

Watered pills are made of fine powder of crude drugs, using water (or yellow rice wine, vinegar, diluted medicinal juice, diluted syrup) as binder.

Pasted pills are made of fine powder of crude drugs, using rice-paste or flour-paste as binder.

Concentrated pills are made of extract or condensed extract of crude drugs, mixing with appropriate excipient or fine powder of crude drugs, using water, honey or honey and water as binders. They may be subdivided into concentrated watered pills, concentrated honeyed pills and concentrated water-honeyed pills, based upon the different binders used in the production.

Wax pill are made of fine powder of crude drugs using wax as a binder.

Micropills are all kinds of pills that is less than 2.5 mm in diameter.

Pills may be classified into kneaded pills, coated pills and dropping pills by the methods of production.

1. General requirement for preparation of pills.

(1) The powdered drugs for pills production should be passed through sieve No.6 or 5, unless otherwise specified.

(2) The honey used for honeyed pills production should be processed before using. According to the degree of processing, it can be divided into primary processed honey, secondary processed and tertiary processed honey, which may be selected and used to prepare honeyed pills, depending on the climate and the varieties of honeyed pills. In preparing big and small honeyed pills by the kneading method, the processed honey should be added to the

drug powder while hot and mixed well, unless otherwise specified. If resin, gum and volatile drugs are contained in the formulation, the processed honey should be added at about 60℃; in preparing water – honeyed pills by water snowball (spray rotating) method, the processed honey should be diluted with boiling water before using.

(3) For preparing concentrated pills the extract or condensed extract should be made by concentrating the decoction and percolate, obtained by decocting and percolating.

(4) Unless otherwise specified, water – honeyed pills, watered pills or concentrated water – honeyed pills, concentrated watered pills should be dried at a temperature below 80℃; pills containing large amount of volatile constituents or starch (including pasted pills) should be dried at a temperature below 60℃. Thermolabile pills should be dried using other proper methods.

(5) Wax used for wax pills should comply with the description under the monograph of the crude drug in the pharmacopoeia. Impurities should be excluded from the wax before using. For production of wax pill, the wax should be heated and melted, cooling to about 60℃, mixed well with drug powders in proportion. The pills should be prepared by the method for honeyed pills while not cool down.

(6) For pills that need to be coated and polished, coat with the coating materials and polish as specified under individual medication.

(7) Pills should be round, integrate and uniform in appearance and colour. Big and small honeyed pills should appear fine, smooth and oily – moistened, with proper hardness. There should be not cracks on the face of wax pills, not wax spots and particles in wax pills.

(8) Pills should be preserved in tightly closed containers.

2. Tests

(1) Determination of water Carry out the method for the determination of water in general (see Ch. P. Appendix). Unless otherwise specified, big honeyed pills, small honeyed pills and concentrated honeyed pills contain not more than 15.0% of water, water – honeyed pills, concentrated water – honeyed pills not more than 12.0%, watered pills, pasted pills and concentrated watered pills not more than 9.0%. The water content in the micro – pills may be determined with the requirements described under each individual pill type. The water content in the wax pills is not required to be tested.

(2) Weight variation Pills to be taken by number are examined by Method 1 and pills to be taken by weight examined by Method 2.

Method 1 Generally, take the largest number of pills in single dosage as one portion (Details stipulated in Ch. P. Appendix). Weigh separately 10 parts and compare with the labelled single or total weight (the largest number of pills in single dosage labelled weight of each pill). The weight variation should comply with the requirements stated in the table below. Not more than 2 parts exceed the limit of weight variation and none doubles the limit of weight variation.

Tab 1

Labelled total weight	Weight variation limit
0.05g or less than 0.05g	±12%
more than 0.05 g to 0.1 g	±11%
more than 0.1 g to 0.3g	±10%
more than 0.3 g to 1.5 g	±9%
more than 1.5 g to 3 g	±8%
more than 3 g to 6 g	±7%
more than 6 g to 9 g	±6%
more than 9 g	±5%

Method 2 Take 10 pills as one part. Weigh separately 10 parts and calculate the average weight, the variation between the weight of each part and the average weight should comply with the requirements stated in the table below. Not more than 2 parts exceed the weight variation limit and none doubles the weight variation limit.

Tab 2

Average weight of one part	Weight variation limit
0.05g or less than 0.05g	±12%
more than 0.05g to 0.1g	±11%
more than 0.1g to 0.3g	±10%
more than 0.3g to 1g	±8%
more than 1g to2g	±7%
more than 2g	±6%

Weight variation of sugar – coated pills should be examined before coating. Pills are not to be sugar – coated until the weight variation of the pill cores complies with the requirements stated in the table above. The weight variation of pills is not examined after sugar – coating.

3. Packing variation The limit of weight variation per pack with pills divided or packed in single should comply with the requirements stated in the table below.

Tab 3

Labelled weight of each pack	Weight variation limit
more than 0.5g to 1g	±11%
more than 1g to 2g	±10%
more than 2g to 3g	±8%
more than 3g to 6g	±6%
more than 6g to 9g	±5%

Procedure Take ten packs of pills and weigh separately the content of each pack (or vial), the variation between the weight and the labelled weight of each pack should comply with the requirement stated in the table above. Not more than 2 packs exceed the weight variation limit and none doubles the weight variation limit.

4. Disintegration test Take 6 pills, select a basket with proper porosity of sieve (for pills with the diameter of less than 2.5mm, 2.5 ~ 3.5mm or more than 3.5mm, using sieves with pores of 0.42 mm, 1 mm or 2 mm in diameter respectively). Carry out the test as described under the disintegration test for tablets, using disk (Ch.P.Appendix). Small honeyed pills, water – honeyed pills and watered pills should be completely disintegrated within 1 hour, and concentrated pills and pasted pills within 2 hours. The disintegration test of micro – pills may be tested with the requirements described under individual monograph, unless otherwise specified. If pills adhere to the disk, thus hindering the determination, take another 6 pills and carry out the determination as described under the disintegration of tablets without disk, pills should be completely disintegrated within the specified time.

In the determination mentioned above, all the pills should pass through the sieve within the specified time. If there are minute granulated masses which cannot pass the sieve but soften without hard core, should be considered to be up to the standard.

No disintegration test is required for big honeyed pills.

Maren Runchang Wan

Maren Runchang Pill[2] is a preparation recorded in the Pharmacopoeia of People's Republic of China. The pill is made of Fructus Cannabis, Semen Armeniacae Amarum, Radix et Rhizoma Rhei, Radix Aucklandiae, Pericarpium Citri Reticulatae, and Radix Paeoniae Alba. It contains sennosides, a cathartic agent and a great quantity of fat.

Description Yellowish – brown big honeyed pills; odor, slightly aromatic; bitter taste, slightly sweet.

Action Catharsis, moisturizing intestine.

Indications Heat stagnated in stomach and intestines, distension in chest and abdomen, constipation.

Usage and dosage 1 ~ 2 pills. 2 times a day.

Precaution Contraindicated in pregnancy.

Specification 6g per pill.

Storage Preserve in tightly closed containers.

Exercise materials

Instruments: balances, beakers, hotplate, screens, scale, blender, pill – forming machine, disintegration apparatus, test unit, etc.

Drugs and reagents: Fructus Cannabis, Semen Armeniacae Amarum (peeled and stir – fried), Radix et Rhizoma Rhei, Radix Aucklandiae, Pericarpium Citri Reticulatae, Radix Paeoniae Alba, etc.

1. Formulation

Fructus Cannabis	120g
Semen Armeniacae Amarum (peeled and stir – fried)	60g
Radix et Rhizoma Rhei	120g
Radix Aucklandiae	60g
Pericarpium Citri Reticulatae	120g
Radix Paeoniae Alba	60g
Process honey	q.s.

2. Procedure

(1) Processing crude drugs: Pulverize the above six ingredients to fine powder, sift through sieve No 5 and mix well.

(2) Making pill mass: To each 100 g of the powder add 140 ~ 160g of tertiary processed honey to make a plastic mass into the proper consistency, neither sticky nor cracking.

(3) Forming pills: Make honeyed pills with the mixed mass in a pill forming machine.

3. Tests

Comply with the general requirements for pills.

Erzhi Wan

Erzhiwan pill[3] is a preparation recorded in the Pharmacopoeia of People's Republic of China. The pill is made of Fructus Ligustri Lucidi (steamed) and Herba Ecliptae. It is produced by condensed extract of part crude drugs, mixing with fine powder of part crude drugs, using honey and water as binders, containing oleanolic acid and polysaccharides.

Description Blackish – brown water – honeyed pills; odour, slight; taste, bitter sweet.

Action To replenish yin of the liver and the kidney and arrest bleeding.

Indications Deficiency of yin of the liver and the kidney marked by dizziness, tinnitus, dryness of the throat and nose, aching of the loins and knees, and excessive menstrual discharge.

Usage and dosage 9g, 2 times a day.

Storage Preserve in well – closed containers, protected from moisture.

Exercise materials

Instruments: funnel, gauze, evaporating dishes, beakers, hotplate, screens, scale, pan, coating pan, and disintegration apparatus test unit, etc.

Drugs and reagents: Fructus Ligustri Lucidi (steamed), Herba Ecliptae, honey, etc.

Exercise methods

1. Formulation

Fructus Ligustri Lucidi (steamed)	500g
Herba Ecliptae	500g
Process honey	60g
Water	q.s.

(A fifth for student's exercise.)

2. Procedure

(1) Processing crude drugs: Pulverize Fructus Ligustri Lucidi to fine powder and sift through sieve No.6. Decoct Herba Ecliptae with water twice for l hour each. Combine the decoctions, filter and evaporate the filtrate appropriately. Add 12 g of processed honey and a quantity of water. Mix well to make binder.

(2) Forming pills by coating method: Mix 3g fine powder of Frtlctus Ligustri Lucidi with a quantity of water to form wet mass with suitable hardness, press through sieve No. 2 to form grains. Rotate the grain in a coating pan to form molds. After being sifted, rotate the molds in the coating pan, spraying the binder, and add fine powders to shape pills.

(3) Forming pills by kneading method: Mix fine powder of Frtlctus Ligustri Lucidi with the binder to form a plastic mass. Prepare sticks and pills from the mass with a pill mold board, knead and rub the pill to round.

(4) Dry pills under 70 ~ 80℃.

3. Tests

Comply with the general requirements for pills, except that the disintegration time is within 2 hours.

Question

Describe the difference between the kneading method and the coating method for produce pills according your experience, especially for Erzhiwan pills.

References

1. Pharmacopoeia Commission of PRC. Pharmacopoeia of P.R.of China (English edition) Volume I. Beijing: Chemical Industry Press. 1997,. 272, 320, Appendix A – 4

2. Pharmacopoeia Commission of PRC. Pharmacopoeia of P.R.of China. Volume I. Beijing: Chemical Industry Press. 2000, 584

3. Pharmacopoeia Commission of PRC. Pharmacopoeia of P.R.of China. Volume I. Beijing: Chemical Industry Press. 2000, 324

实验七　栓　　剂

【实验目的】

1．熟悉栓剂基质的分类、特点及适用情况。

2．掌握熔融法制备栓剂的方法。

【实验指导】

中药栓剂[1]系指中药提取物或中药粉末与适宜的基质混合制成具有一定形状和重量以供直肠、阴道、或其他人体腔道给药的固体制剂。它可发挥局部或全身治疗作用。目前常用的有肛门栓和阴道栓。

1．栓剂生产和储藏的一般要求

(1) 栓剂一般使用的基质有下列两类：

油脂性基质：如天然的可可豆脂，半合成的脂肪酸甘油酯等。该类基质一般常温时为固体，利于成型，便于施入腔道，体温时迅速融化，释放内部药物。水溶性基质：如甘油、明胶、水的比例混合物，聚乙二醇，泊洛沙姆等。该类基质体温下一般不熔融，能缓缓溶于体液而释放药物。在基质中也可以加入适宜的表面活性剂以促进药物的释放和被机体吸收。

(2) 供栓剂用的固体药物，一般应预先用适宜的方法制成细粉或最细粉。根据施用的腔道和使用目的的不同，制成合适的形状。

(3) 栓剂中的药物与基质应混合均匀。其外形应光滑，无刺激性，并且有适宜的硬度；塞入腔道后，应能融化、软化或溶解，并与分泌液混合，释放药物，产生局部或全身的作用。

(4) 栓剂使用的内包装材料应无毒性，并不得与药物和基质发生理化反应。

(5) 栓剂一般应在30℃以下密闭保存，防止受热、受潮。

2．栓剂的检查

(1) 重量差异　取供试品10粒，精密称定总重量，求出平均粒重，再分别精密称定每一粒重，计算每一粒重量与标示粒重（无标示重量，则取平均重量）之比。1g或小于1g栓剂，重量差异为±10%；1～3g栓剂重量差异限度为±7.5%；3g以上栓剂，重量差异限度为±5.0%。超出限度的粒不得多于1粒，并不得超出限度一倍。

(2) 融变时限　按《中国药典》融变时限检查法，取供试品3粒，在室温放置1小时后，分别放在3个金属架的下层圆板上，装入各自的套筒内，并用挂钩固定。除另有规定外，将上述装置分别垂直浸入盛有不少于4L的37.0±0.5℃水的容器中，其上端位置应在水面下90mm处。容器中装一转动器，每隔10min在水中翻转该装置一次。

结果判断　除另有规定外，脂肪性基质的栓剂3粒均应在30min内全部融化、软化，或触压时无硬心；水溶性基质的栓剂3粒应在60min内全部溶解。如有1粒不合格，应另取3粒复试，均应符合规定。

实验　双黄连栓（小儿消炎栓）

双黄连栓（Shuanghuanglian Shuan）收载于2000年版药典一部[2]。本方由金银花（忍冬 *Lonicera japonica* Thunb.，红腺忍冬 *L. hypoglauca* Miq.，山银花 *L. confusa* DC.，或毛花柱忍冬 *L. dasystyla* Rehd. 的花）、黄芩（黄芩 *Scutellaria baicalensis* Georgi 的根）、连翘（连翘 *Forsythia suspense*（Thunb.）Vahl 的果实）组成。金银花主要含绿原酸、木犀草素、异绿原酸等。2000年版药典金银花的定量成份为绿原酸；黄芩主要含黄芩苷，黄芩素，汉黄芩素等。黄芩的定量指标为黄芩苷。连翘主要含齐墩果酸，连翘酚，连翘苷等。连翘苷为连翘的定量成分。2000年版药典小儿消炎栓以黄芩苷、绿原酸为定性指标。以黄芩苷为定量指标。

性状：本品为棕色或深棕色的栓剂

功能主治：清热解毒，轻宣风热，用于外感风热，发热，咳嗽，咽痛，上呼吸道感染，肺炎。

规格：每粒重1.5g。

用法和剂量：直肠给药，小儿每次1粒，每日2～3次。

贮藏：密封，置阴凉干燥处。

【实验材料】

仪器：肛门栓模、电炉、水浴锅、不锈钢锅、蒸发皿、烧杯（250ml、500ml、1000ml）、抽滤装置、干燥箱、天平、波美比重计、酒精比重计、100ml量筒等，以及一套栓剂融变时限检查仪器。

材料：金银花、黄芩、连翘、半合成脂肪酸甘油酯（36型）、甘油、软肥皂、90%乙醇、乙醇、2mol/L HCl溶液、40%NaOH液、pH试纸（1～14）。

【实验方法】

1．处方

金银花	2500g
黄芩	2500g
连翘	5000g
半合成脂肪酸甘油酯	780g

制成肛门栓1000粒

（学生实验可采用百分之一量）

2．制法：

（1）黄芩提取与精制

取黄芩药材25g，分别加水250ml、200ml煎煮2次，第一次1小时，第二次0.5小时，合并两次煎液，过滤，滤液浓缩至100ml，在80℃下，用2mol/L HCl液调pH 1～2，搅拌均匀，静止24小时，滤过，沉淀物加6～8倍水，用40%的NaOH溶液调pH 7.0～7.5，加入等量乙醇，搅拌使溶解，滤过，滤液再用2mol/L HCl溶液，调pH 2.0，搅拌均匀，静止 12 小时，滤过，收集沉淀，得黄芩苷粗提取物。

(2) 金银花，连翘提取与精制

取金银花 25g，连翘 50g 分别加水 750ml、600ml 煎煮 2 次，第一次 1 小时，第二次 0.5 小时，合并滤液，过滤，滤液浓缩至相对密度 1.20～1.25（70～80℃），浸膏冷至 40℃，缓慢加入乙醇使含醇量达 75%，静止 12 小时，滤取上清液回收乙醇至无醇味，再将浓缩液加入乙醇使含醇量达 85%，搅拌充分，静止 12 小时，滤取上清液，回收乙醇至无醇味，得提取物。

(3) 样品浓缩与干燥

将黄芩苷粗提取物加入到金银花与连翘提取物中，搅拌均匀（如需要加少量水混匀），调 pH 7.0～7.5，减压浓缩成稠膏状，真空干燥，粉碎成细粉（100 目）。

(4) 熔化法制备栓剂

取半合成脂肪酸甘油酯 8g 于蒸发皿中，水浴（80℃）加热熔化均匀，将温度保持在 40℃以上，加入上述干膏细粉，充分搅拌混合均匀，在栓模内壁，涂上水性润滑剂之后，将融熔状态的样品，缓缓倾注于模孔中，放冷，完全凝固，成型后削去溢出部分，起模，包装，即可。

【思考题】

1. 小儿消炎栓是起局部作用还是起全身作用？为何选脂肪酸甘油酯为基质？

2. 简要说明黄芩提取与精制每一步的操作目的？

参 考 文 献

1. 国家药典委员会.《中华人民共和国药典》一部. 北京：化学工业出版社. 2000，附录.

2. 国家药典委员会.《中华人民共和国药典》一部. 北京：化学工业出版社. 2000，419

Exercise 7 Suppositories

Learning objectives

1. Learn classification, characteristics and uses of bases applied in suppositories.
2. Practice and learn the preparation of suppositories with melting method.

Instruction

TCM suppositories[1-2] are solid preparation made by incorporating extracts of crude drugs or powdered crude drugs in suitable bases, intended for introduction into the cavities, such as rectal and vaginal, of the human body. It can exert local or systemic effects.

1. The general requirements of production and storage of suppositories:

(1) The bases for suppositories are usually divided into the lipid base, such as cocoa butter, and semi-synthetic fatty glycerides, etc., and the water-soluble base, such as a mixture of glycerin and gelatin, PEG, and poloxamer, etc. The lipid base is generally solid at room temperature, easy to be moulded and convenient for introduction into the cavities of the body, and rapidly melt and release drug at body temperature. The water-soluble-bases may not melt at body temperature. When the suppository with a water-soluble-base is introduced into the cavity of human body, it is miscible with body fluid to release the medicaments gradually.

(2) Generally solid drug substances should be made into fine or very fine powders before use. Suppositories are made in a suitable shape to the place of entry into the body.

(3) The drug substance and bases in suppositories should be mixed well. Suppositories should be smooth in appearance and non-irritating with appropriate hardness. They can melt, soften, or dissolve when inserted in the cavity, and are miscible with body fluid to release drug substance and exert topical and systemic effect.

(4) The immediate packing materials for suppositories should be non-toxic and do not interact physicochemically with the medicaments or bases in the suppositories.

(5) Generally suppositories should be stored closely at a temperature below 30℃ and protected from heat and moisture.

2. Tests

(1) Weight variation　Weigh together 10 suppositories and determine average weight.

Then weigh individually each of the 10 suppositories. Compare the weight of each suppository with the labelled weight (If no labelled weight is stated, compare the weight of each suppository with the average weight calculated). Weight variation is limited in respectively,

± 10%, ± 7.5%, and ± 5.0%, for each labelled weight in less 1.0g, 1.0 ~ 3.0g, and more than 3.0g.

(2) Disintegration test According as the specified method for the disintegration test in the Pharmacopoeia of the People's Republic of China, take 3 of the suppositories being examined and allow them to stand at room temperature for 1 hour. Place them on the lower discs of 3 metal devices respectively. Then insert the devices into separate sleeves and fix them by means of hooks unless otherwise specified. Place each piece of the above apparatus in 3 vessels separately. Each containing not less than 4 litres of water at 37.0℃ ± 0.5℃ and fitted with a slow stirrer and a means of holding the apparatus vertically 90mm below the surface of water. After each 10 minutes invert each apparatus without allowing it to emerge from the liquid.

Interpretation: Unless otherwise specified, all of the fat – based suppositories should disintegrate, soften, or have no solid core offer resistance to pressure, in not more than 30 minutes; all of the water – soluble based suppositories should completely dissolve in not more than 60 minutes. If one of the suppositories fails to comply with the requirements, repeat the test on 3 additional suppositories and all of them should comply with the requirements.

Shuanghuanglian Suppository

Shuanghuanglian suppositories[3-4] is collected in the Pharmacopeia of the people's Republic of China, Volume I (2000). The drug product is prepared from flos lonicerae (flowers of *Lonicera japonica* Thunb., *L. hypoglauca* Miq., *L. confusa* DC., or *L. dasystyla* Rehd.), fructus forsythiae (fruits of *Forsythia suspense* (Thunb.) Vahl), and radix scutellariae (roots of *Scutellaria baicalensis* Georgi). Chlorogenil acid, baicalin, and phillyrin are the major constituents of Flos lonicerae, radix scutellariae, and fructus forsythiae for assay of the three crude drugs described in the Chinese Pharmacopeia, respectively.

Description Brown or dark brown suppository.

Action To remove heat and counteract toxicity to dispel wind.

Indication Affected by wind – heat, fever, cough sore throat, infection of upper respiratory tract, pneumonia.

Specification 1.5g per suppository.

Usage and dosage 1 suppository, 2 ~ 3 times a day, to be administrated through rectal.

Storage Preserve in well closed container. Stored in a cool and dry place.

Exercise materials

Instruments: suppository moulds, hotplate, water – bath, stainless steel pot, evaporating dish, beaker (250ml, 500ml, and 1000ml), filter apparatus, dry oven, balance, alcohol densimeter, Baume hydrometer, measuring cylinder (100ml), and a set of apparatus for suppository disintegration test.

Materials: Flos lonicerae, fructus forsythiae, radix scutellariae, semi – synthetic fatty glycerides (36 type), glycerin, soft – soap, alcohol, 2mol/L Hydrochloric acid, 40% sodium hydroxide, and pH – indicate paper (1 ~ 14).

Exercise method

1. Formulation

Flos Lonicerae	2500g
Fructus Forsythiae	5000g
Radix Scutellarie	2500g
Semi – synthetic fatty glycerides	780g

made up into 1000 suppositories

One percent for student's exercise

2. preparation

(1) Extracting and refining for Radix Scutellariae:

Decoct 25g of Radix Scutellariae with 250 ~ 200 ml of water 2 times, 1 hour for the first time and half an hour for the second time. Combine the decoction, filter and concentrate to a quantity about 100ml, Add 2mol/L Hydrochloric acid to the concentrated decoction at 80℃ to adjust pH value to 1.0 – 2.0 to stir even. Let it stand for 24 hours and filter. Add 6 – 8 volumes of water to the precipitate, add 40% sodium hydroxide to adjust pH value 7.0 ~ 7.5, then add a same volume of ethanol, stir to dissolve and filter. Add 2mol/L of hydrochloric acid to adjust the pH value of the filtrate to 2.0, stir it to even, set on still for 12 hours and filter, to obtain a coarse extraction of radix scutellariae.

(2) Extracting and refining for flos lonicerae and fructus forsythiae.

Decoct 25g of flos lonicerae and 50g of fructus forsythiae with 750 ~ 600ml of water for twice, 1 hour for the first time and 0.5 hour for the second time. Combine the decoctions and concentrate to a relative density of 1.20 ~ 1.25 (70 ~ 80℃), to obtain a liquid extract. After cooling to 40℃, slowly add ethanol under stirring till a content of ethanol to 75%, stand for 12 hours. Separate the supernate and recover from ethanol. Add ethanol again to the concentrated extract, make the content of ethanol to 85%, stir well, let it stand for 12 hours, separate the supernate recover ethanol to no ethanolic smell, to obtain a liquid extraction.

(3) Concentrating and drying

Mix the above coarse extracts obtained. Stir well and adjust the pH value to 7.0 – 7.5, concentrate under reduced pressure to a thick extract, dry under a lower temperature to completely drying, pulverize to fine powder (100 mesh).

(4) Preparation of suppository with a melt method.

Take semi – synthetic fatty glycerides 8g, heat to melt in a water bath. Keep temperature at 40℃ ± 2℃, add the above dried extract fine powder, mix well and pour slowly into moulds to make into 10 suppositories. Cooling and modeling, take out and pack.

Questions

1. Do the suppository exert either local or systemic effects? Why is semi – synthetic fatty glycerides selected for the suppositories' base?

2. What scientific principles are the extraction process of radix scutellariae based on?

References

1. Pharmacopoeia Commission of PRC, Pharmacopoeia of the People's Republic of China Volume I. Beijing: Chemical Industry Press. 2000, Appendix 18.

2. Pharmacopoeia Commission of PRC, Pharmacopoeia of the People's Republic of China (English edition), Volume I. Beijing: Chemical Industry Press. 1997, Appendix A – 13

3. Pharmacopoeia Commission of PRC, Pharmacopoeia of the People's Republic of China (English edition), Volume I. Beijing: Chemical Industry Press. 1997, 407

4. Pharmacopoeia Commission of PRC, Pharmacopoeia of the People's Republic of China. Volume I, Beijing: Chemical Industry Press. 2000, 419

实验八　颗　粒　剂

【实验目的】

1．熟悉中药颗粒剂的质量要求。

2．掌握中药颗粒剂的一般制法。

【实验指导】

颗粒剂[1]系指药材提取物与适宜的辅料或药材细粉制成的颗粒状制剂，分为可溶性颗粒剂、混悬性颗粒剂和泡腾性颗粒剂。

1．颗粒剂生产与贮藏的一般要求

(1) 配制颗粒剂时可加入适宜的辅料、矫味剂和芳香剂。

(2) 除另有规定外，药材应按各该品种项下规定的方法进行提取、纯化、浓缩至规定相对密度的清膏，喷雾制粒或喷雾干燥，制成细粉，加适量的辅料，混匀，制成颗粒；或加适量的辅料或药材细粉，与浓缩的浸膏混匀，制成颗粒，干燥。辅料用量应予以控制，一般前者不超过干膏量的2倍，后者不超过清膏量的5倍。

(3) 挥发油应均匀喷入干燥颗粒中，密闭至规定时间；或采用保护性技术加入挥发油。

(4) 颗粒剂应干燥、颗粒均匀、色泽一致，无吸潮、软化、结块、潮解等现象。

(5) 除另有规定外，颗粒剂应密封贮藏。

2．颗粒剂的检查

(1) 粒度　照粒度测定法（见《中华人民共和国药典》附录）检查。不能通过一号筛和能通过五号筛的颗粒和粉末总和，不得过15%。

(2) 水分　照水分测定法（《中华人民共和国药典》附录）测定。除另有规定外，不得过6.0%。

测定用的供试品，一般先破碎成直径不超过3mm的颗粒或碎片。

第一法（烘干法）本法适用于不含或少含挥发性成分的药品。取供试品2～5g，平铺于干燥至恒重的扁形称瓶中，厚度不超过5mm，疏松供试品不超过10mm，精密称定，打开瓶盖在100～105℃干燥5小时，将瓶盖盖好，移置干燥器中，冷却30分钟，精密称定重量，再在上述温度干燥1小时，冷却，称重，至连续两次称重的差异不超过5mg为止。根据减失的重量，计算供试品中含水量（%）。

其它方法参见《中华人民共和国药典》一部附录。

(3) 溶化性　取供试品1袋（多剂量包装者取10g)，加热水200ml，搅拌5分钟，立即观察。颗粒剂应全部溶化或混悬。泡腾性颗粒剂遇水时应立即产生二氧化碳气并呈泡腾状。颗粒剂均不得有焦屑等异物。

(4) 装量差异　单剂量分装的颗粒剂装量差异限度应符合表中规定。

检查法　取供试品10袋（瓶），分别称定每袋（瓶）内容物的重量，每袋（瓶）的重量与标示装量相比较（凡无标示装量应与平均装量相比较），超出限度的不得多于 2 袋（瓶），并不得有 1 袋（瓶）超出限度一倍。

多剂量分装的颗粒剂照最低装量检查法（《中华人民共和国药典》附录）检查，应符合规定。

装量差异限度

标示装量	装量差异限度
1.0g 或 1.0g 以下	±10%
1.0g 以上至 1.5g	±8%
1.5g 以上至 6g	±7%
6g 以上	±5%

（5）微生物限度　照微生物限度检查法（《中华人民共和国药典》附录）检查，应符合规定。

实验　板蓝根颗粒

板蓝根颗粒[2]（Banlangen Keli）是《中华人民共和国药典》收载的中药制剂。本品为中药板蓝根制成的颗粒剂。板蓝根为十字花科植物菘蓝 *Isatis indigotica* Fort. 的干燥根。主含靛蓝（indigotin）、靛玉红（indirubin）、β－谷甾醇（β－sitosterol）、γ－谷甾醇（γ－sitosterol）以及多种氨基酸。还含黑芥子苷（sinigrin）、靛苷（indoxyl－β－glucoside）等成分。

性状：本品为棕色或棕褐色的颗粒；味甜、微苦或味微苦（无糖型）。

功能与主治：清热解毒，凉血利咽，消肿。用于热毒壅盛，咽喉肿痛；扁桃腺炎，腮腺炎见上述证候者。

用法与用量：开水冲服，一次 5～10g（含糖型）或 3～6g（无糖型），一日 3～4 次。

规格：每袋装（1）5g；（2）10g。

贮藏：密封。

【实验材料】

仪器：电炉、普通天平、铝锅、比重瓶、烧瓶（1000ml，500ml）、药筛、瓷盘、紫外灯等。

药品和试剂：板蓝根、乙醇、蔗糖、糊精、滤纸、茚三酮试液等。

【实验方法】

1．处方

板蓝根	1400g
糖粉	Q.S.
糊精	Q.S.
制成 1000g	

2．制法

（1）提取与浓缩　取板蓝根 50g，加水煎煮二次，第一次 2 小时，第二次 1 小时，合并煎液，滤过，滤液浓缩至相对密度为1.20（50℃）。

（2）精制　取浓缩液加乙醇使含醇量为60%，搅匀，静置使沉淀，取上清液回收乙醇，浓缩至适量，得清膏。

（3）制颗粒　取清膏1份、蔗糖2份、糊精1.3份，制成颗粒，干燥，即得。

3．检查

应符合颗粒剂有关的要求。

4．鉴别

（1）取本品0.5g，加水5ml使溶解，静置，取上清液点于滤纸上，晾干，置紫外光灯（365nm）下观察，显蓝紫色。

（2）取本品0.5g，加水10ml使溶解，滤过，取滤液1ml，加茚三酮试液0.5ml，置水浴中加热数分钟，显蓝紫色。

实验　抗感颗粒

抗感颗粒[3]（Kanggan Keli）是《中华人民共和国药典》收载的中药制剂。金银花为忍冬科植物忍冬 *Lonicera japonica* Thunb.、红腺忍冬 *Lonicera hypoglauca* Miq.、山银花 *Lonicera confusa* DC. 或毛花柱忍冬 *Lonicera dasystyla* Rehd. 的干燥花蕾或带初开的花。金银花具清热解毒、凉散风热的功效，主要含绿原酸（chlorogenic acid）、异绿原酸（isochlorogenic acid）和挥发油。赤芍为毛茛科植物芍药 *Paeonia lactiflora* Pall. 或川芍药 *Paeonia veitchii* Lynch 的干燥根，具清热凉血、散瘀止痛的功效，主要含芍药苷（paeoniflorin）。绵马贯众为鳞毛蕨科植物粗茎鳞毛蕨 *Dryopterix crassirhizoma* Nakai 的干燥根茎及叶柄残基，主要含绵马酸（filixic acid）BBB、PBB、PBP等，黄绵马酸（flavaspidic acid）AB、BB、PB以及白绵马素 albaspidin，还含东北贯众素 dryocrassin 及三萜成分。

性状：本品为黄棕色的颗粒；味甜、微苦。

功能与主治：清热解毒。用于外感风热引起的发热，头痛，鼻塞，喷嚏，咽痛，全身乏力，酸痛等症。

用法与用量：开水冲服，一次10g，一日3次；小儿酌减或遵医嘱。

规格：每袋装10g。

贮藏：密封。

【实验材料】

仪器：电炉、普通天平、煎药锅、比重瓶、烧瓶（1000ml，500ml，100ml）、药筛、瓷盘、紫外灯、微量点样器、层析缸等。

材料：金银花、赤芍、绵马贯众、乙醇、蔗糖、糊精、硅胶G薄层板、乙酸乙酯、甲醇、甲酸等。

【实验方法】

1．处方

金银花　　210g

赤芍　　　　　　　　210g

绵马贯众　　　　　　70g

2．制法

（1）提取与浓缩　取以上三味十分之一量，加水煎煮二次，每次 1.5 小时，合并滤液，滤过，滤液浓缩至 25ml。

（2）精制　取浓缩液加乙醇使含醇量为 50%，搅匀，放置过夜，滤过，滤液回收乙醇，并浓缩至相对密度为 1.28～1.30（50℃）的清膏。

（3）制颗粒　取清膏 1 份，蔗糖粉 1.65 份，糊精 1.5 份及乙醇适量，制成颗粒，干燥，即得。

3．检查

应符合颗粒剂有关的要求。

4．鉴别

取本品 4g，研细，加醋酸乙酯 15ml，置水浴上回流提取 1 小时，放冷，滤过，滤液蒸干。残渣加甲醇 1ml 使溶解，作为供试品溶液。另取绿原酸对照品，加甲醇制成每 1ml 含 1mg 的溶液，作为对照品溶液。照《中国药典》附录薄层色谱法试验，吸取供试品溶液 10μl、对照品溶液 2μl，分别点于同一以羟甲基纤维素钠为黏合剂的硅胶 G 薄层板上，以醋酸丁酯－甲酸－水（14∶5∶5）的上层溶液为展开剂，展开，取出，晾干，置紫外光灯（365nm）下检视。供试品色谱中，在与对照品色谱相应的位置上，显相同颜色的荧光斑点。

【思考题】

1．请叙述颗粒剂的质量要求有哪些？

2．请说明蔗糖、糊精、乙醇在制备颗粒剂中的作用。

参　考　文　献

1．中华人民共和国药典委员会．中华人民共和国药典（一部）．北京：化学工业出版社．2000，附录 7

2．中华人民共和国药典委员会．中华人民共和国药典（一部）．北京：化学工业出版社．2000，163，490

3．中华人民共和国药典委员会．中华人民共和国药典（一部）．北京：化学工业出版社．2000，125，177，271，474

Exercise 8 Granules

Exercise objectives

1. Practice and learn the general process to produce medicinal granules made from crude drugs.

2. Understand the characteristics and the quality control of the granules.

Instruction

Granules[1-2] are made of extracts or fine powders of crude drugs and suitable excipients with granular forms. They are classified into soluble, suspensible, or effervescent granule products.

1. The general requirements of production and storage of medicinal granules

(1) Proper excipients, flavoring agents, aromatic and colouring agents may be added in preparation of granules.

(2) The crude drugs should be processed by extraction, purification and concentration to form an extract with a required relative density. The extract is then spray – granulated or spray – dried to fine powder particles, add a quantity of excipients, mix well to make granules; or add a quantity of excipients or finely powdered crude drugs into the concentrated extract, and mix well, granulate and then dry the granules. The amount of excipients added is not more than 2 times of that of dried extract. or not more than 5 times of that of the thin extract.

(3) The volatile oil should be sprayed evenly upon dried granules stored in well – closed containers for the required time, unless a technique for protection is applied.

(4) Medicinal granules, should be dry, uniform in appearance and colour, without moisture absorption and softening.

(5) Medicinal granules should be stored in tightly closed containers.

2. Tests

(1) Size of granules Test with the granulometry method stipulated in Ch.P. Appendix. The total granules and powders which cannot pass through sieve No.1 and pass through sieve No.5 are not more than 15%.

(2) Determination of water Carry out the method for the determination of water (Ch.P.Appendix). The medicinal granules contain not more than 6.0% of water unless specified otherwise.

Method I (Drying in oven method)

The method is used for the determination of water in crude drugs containing no, or scarcely any volatile constituents. Place 2 – 5g of substance being examined in flat weighing bottle, previously dried to constant weight, to form a smooth layer not exceeding 5 mm in thickness, or not exceeding 10 mm in thickness for substance of loose texture and then weight accurately. Dry in an oven at 100 ~ 105℃ for 5 hours with the stopper of the bottle removed. Upon opening the oven, close the bottle promptly and allow it to cool in a desiccator for 30 minutes. Weigh accurately and dry it again under similar condition for 1 hour, cool and weigh. Repeat the operation until the difference between two successive weighings is not more than 5 mg. Calculate the percentage content of water in the substance being examined according the weight loss on drying.

The other methods may be used. Please see the Chinese Pharmacopoeia.

(3) Determination of dispersibility To 1 pack (10g for granules presented in multi – dose) of medicinal granules, 200ml of hot water, stir for 5 minutes. Granules should be completely dissolved or suspended in water evenly; effervescent granules should produce carbon dioxide bubbles and be in effervescent state immediately when they meet with water. All kinds of granules should not show any foreign matter, such as burned charrings and so on.

(4) Weight variation The weight variation limit of single dose Package of medicinal granules should comply with the requirements stated in the table below.

Labelled weight per pack	Weight variation limit
1.0g or less than 1.0g	± 10%
more than 1.0g to 1.5g	± 8%
more than 1.5 g to 6 g	± 7%
more than 6 g	± 5%

Procedure Take 10 packs of medicinal granules and weigh the individual content of each pack. Compare the weight of each pack with the labelled amount (if no labeled weight is stated, compare weight of each pack with the average weight calculated). Not more than 2 packs in weight variation exceed the weight variation limit stated in the table above and none doubles the limit.

Packing variation for granules presented in multi – dose should comply with the test for minimum fill (Ch. P. Appendix).

(5) Microbial limit test Comply with the requirements stated under microbial limit test (Ch. P. Appendix).

Banlangen Granules

Banlangen Granules[3] are the granules prepared from Radix Isatidis. It is recorded in the pharmacopoeia of PRC. Radix Isatidis is the dried root of *Isatis indigotica* Fort. It contains many constituents such as indigotin, indirubin, β – sitosterol, γ – sitosterol and multiplicate amino acids.

Description Brown granules; taste, sweet, slightly bitter.

Action To remove toxic heat, to reduce heat in blood and be beneficial for throat, detumescence.

Indication Sore and tumid throat with pyretic toxicity; tonsillitis and parotitis with the above symptoms.

Use and dosage 5 ~ 10g, 3 ~ 4 times a day.

Specification 5g or 10g per bag.

Storage Preserve in tightly closed containers.

Exercise materials

Instrument: electric cooker, scale, aluminium boiler, flask (1000ml, 500ml), sieve, porcelain plate, ultraviolet light. etc.

Drugs and Reagents: Radix Isatidis, ethanol, sucrose, dextrin, filter paper, ninhydrin TS etc.

Exercise method

1. Formulation

Radix Isatidis	1400g
sucrose	Q.S.
dextrin	Q.S.

Make 1000g of granules.

2. Procedure

(1) Extraction and concentration Decoct 50g of Radix Isatidis with water twice, 2 hours for the first time and 1 hour for the second time. Combine the decoctions and filter. Concentrate the filtrate to an extract with a relative density of 1.20 (50℃).

(2) Refinement Adjust the concentration of ethanol to 60%, stir well, and let stand to precipitate completely. Recover ethanol of the supernatant and concentrate to an appropriate quantity.

(3) Making granules Make granules with 1 portion of the extract, 2 portions of sucrose, 1.3 portions of dextrin and a quantity of ethanol, and dry.

3. Tests

Comply with the requirements of granules.

4. Identification

(1) Dissolve 0.5g of the granules in 5ml of water, stand. Apply the supernatant to a

piece of filter paper, dry it in air, and examine under ultraviolet light (365nm); a bluish - purple colour is shown.

(2) Dissolve 0.5g of the granules in 10ml of water, and filter. To 1ml of the filtrate, add 0.5ml of ninhydrin TS, heat in a water bath for several minutes; a bluish - purple colour is produced.

Kanggan Granules

Kanggan Granules[4] are recorded in Pharmacopoeia of PRC. Honeysuckle Flower (Flos Lonicerae) is the dried flower bud or opening flower of *Lonicera japonica* Thunb., *Lonicera hypoglauca* Miq., *Lonicera confusa* DC. or *Lonicera dasystyla* Rehd. (Fam. Caprifoliaceae. It contains chlorogenic acid, isochlorogenic acid and volatile oils. Red Peony Root (Radix Paeoniae Rubra) is the dried root of *Paeonia lactiflora* Pall., *Paeonia veitchii* Lynch (Fam. Ranunculaceae. It contains paeoniflorin. Male Fern Rhizome (Rhizoma Dryopteris Crassirhizomae) is the dried rhizome and frond bases of *Dryopterix crassirhizoma* Nakai (Fam. Dryopteridaceae. It contains filixic acid BBB、PBB、PBP, flavaspidic acid AB、BB、PB, albaspidin, dryocrassin and triterpenes.

Description Yellowish - brown granules; taste, sweet, slightly bitter.

Action To remove heat and counteract toxicity.

Use and dosage 10g, 3 times a day, taken with boiled water. Appropriately reduce the dosage for children or follow physician's advice.

Specification 10g per bag.

Storage Preserve in tightly closed containers.

Exercise materials

Instrument: Hotplate, scale, decoction pan, flask (1000ml, 500ml, 100ml, sieve, porcelain plate, ultraviolet detector, micro - syringes for TLC, TLC developing chamber, etc.

Drugs and reagents: Flos Lonicerae, Radix Paeoniae Rubra, Rhizoma Dryopteris Crassirhizomae, ethanol, sucrose, dextrin, silica gel G plate, butyl acetate, formic acid, methanol etc.

Exercise method

1. Ingredients

Flos Lonicerae	210g
Radix Paeoniae Rubra	210g
Rhizoma Dryopteris Crassirhizomae	70g

2. Procedure

(1) Extraction and concentration Decoct the above three ingredients twice for 1.5 hours each, combine the decoctions, filter, concentrate the filtrate to 25ml.

(2) Refinement Add ethanol to produce a solution containing 50% of ethanol, stir well, stand overnight, filter, concentrate the filtrate to a thin extract with a relative density of 1.28 ~ 1.30 (50℃).

(3) Making granules Make granules with 1 portion of the extract, 1.65 portions of sucrose, 1.5 portions of dextrin and a quantity of ethanol, and dry.

3. Tests

Comply with the requirements of granules.

4. Identification

To 4g, finely powdered, add 15ml of ethyl acetate, heat under reflux in a water bath for 1 hour, cool, and filter. Evaporate the filtrate to dryness, and dissolve the residue in 1ml of methanol as the test solution. Dissolve chlorogenic acid CRS in methanol to produce a solution containing 1mg per ml as the reference solution. Carry out the method for thin layer chromatography (Ch.P.Appendix), using silica gel G containing sodium carboxymethyl cellulose as the coating substance and the upper layer of butyl acetate – formic acid – water (14:5:5) as the mobile phase. Apply separately 10μl of the solution and 2μl of the reference solution to the plate. After developing and removal of the plate, dry it in air. Examine under ultraviolet light (365nm), the fluorescent spot in the chromatogram obtained with the test solution corresponds in position and colour to the spot in the chromatogram obtained with the reference solution.

Questions

1. Describe the quality requirements of granules.
2. What roles did the ethanol, sucrose, and dextrin act in production of the granules?

Reference

1. Pharmacopoeia Commission of PRC. Pharmacopoeia of the People's Republic of China (volume 1). Beijing: Chemical industry press, 2000, Appendix 7, 163, 490, 125, 177, 271, 474

2. Pharmacopoeia Commission of PRC. Pharmacopoeia of the People's Republic of China (volume 1). Beijing: Chemical industry press. English edition 1997, Appendix I A – 5

3. Pharmacopoeia Commission of PRC. Pharmacopoeia of the People's Republic of China (volume 1). Beijing: Chemical industry press. English edition 1997, 243

4. Pharmacopoeia Commission of PRC. Pharmacopoeia of the People's Republic of China (volume 1). Beijing: Chemical industry press. English edition 1997, 312

实验九　片　　剂

【实验目的】

1．熟悉片剂制备的基本工艺过程。
2．掌握片剂质量检查方法。
3．了解压片机的基本要求和结构。

【实验指导】

片剂[1]系指药物与适宜的辅料通过制剂技术制成圆片状或其他形式的片状制剂，为最常用的制剂剂型之一。中药或天然药物片剂可以由药材细粉、药材提取物、药材提取物加药材细粉或从药材中提取精制的有效成分与适宜辅料混匀压制而成的，分为药材全粉片、浸膏、半浸膏片以及用有效成分制成的片剂。根据使用途径可分为口服片剂、口腔用片剂及其他途径应用的片剂。片剂的制备方法有直接压片、干法制粒压片和湿法制粒压片。

1．制备片剂的一般要求

(1) 原料药与辅料应混合均匀。小剂量或含有毒剧药物的片剂，可根据药物的性质用适宜的方法使药物分散均匀。

(2) 凡属挥发性或遇热分解的药物，在制片过程中应避免受热损失。制片的颗粒应控制水分，以适应制片工艺的需要，并防止片剂在贮藏期间发霉、变质、失效。

(3) 凡具有不适的臭和味、刺激性、易潮解或遇光易变质的药物，制成片剂后可包糖衣或薄膜衣。对一些遇胃液易破坏、刺激胃黏膜或需要在肠内释放的药物，制成片剂后可包肠溶衣。为适应阴道局部用的需要，可制成阴道用片剂。有些药物也可根据需要制成泡腾片、含片、咀嚼片等。

(4) 片剂外观应完整光洁，色泽均匀；应有适宜的硬度，以免在包装、贮运过程中发生碎片。

(5) 片剂一般应密封贮藏。

2．湿法制粒

除挥发性及对湿、热不稳定的药物之外，多数药物均可采用湿法制粒压片。

湿法制粒一般过程如下：

(1) 将原料和辅料粉末称重后充分混合。小剂量或含毒剧药的片剂，可根据药物的性质，采用适当的方法使药物分散均匀。

(2) 制备制粒溶液：润湿剂或黏合剂。

(3) 将粉末和制粒液捏合成合适黏度的软材（软材软硬适当，即手握成团，轻压能散）。

(4) 将软材用筛网或湿法制粒机压迫通过制粒。

(5) 将颗粒用烘箱或流化床干燥。应根据药料的性质，选用适宜的温度及时间干燥。颗粒中的水分应适应工艺需要，并防止成品在贮存期内潮解、霉变或失效。

（6）将干燥的颗粒用筛网整成合适的大小以备压片。

（7）将润滑剂（和崩解剂）与颗粒混合，经检验合格后压片。挥发性药物的加入除采用喷入法外，可制成微囊、环糊精包合后混入颗粒压片。

3．压片机

压片机是片剂生产的关键设备。旋转式压片机和高速旋转式压片机具有产量高，质量稳定的特点，已经成为主流产品。先进的高速旋转式压片机为全封闭结构，用不锈钢制成，以保持内部清洁并与外部隔离，并有清除不合格产品的自动系统。其吸尘设备可清除残留物和生产中的浮尘。生产能力每小时可达二十多万片。制剂实验室常用的压片机为单冲压片机。

（1）TDP 单冲压片机

本机用以将各种颗粒状原料压成圆片，是一种小型台式电动连续压片的机器，也可以手摇。适合于实验室实验和小规模生产。该机只可装一付冲模，物料的充填深度、压片厚度均可调节。最大压片压力 1.5 千牛；最大压片直径 12 毫米；最大充填深度 11 毫米；最大片剂厚度 6 毫米；生产能力 6000 片/小时。

（2）ZDY8 重型单冲压片机

本机可应用于医药实验室、化工、食品、以及其他相关行业，可连续压制异型、各种圆形的片状物，并可在双面刻字和简单标志。本机特别适用于小批量生产。

本机配最大压力 8 吨，最大压片直径 18 毫米，最大生产能力 5400 片/小时。

（3）安装和使用单冲压片机注意事项

①安装下冲。

②固定模圈在模板上，调节片重调节器和出片调节器。

③安装上冲，调节压力调节器，用手动轮，使得上冲下降到模圈孔穴的中心位置。

④将压片用料装入饲料靴和料斗。用手转动轮试压，收集产品试样。

⑤用手指压碎试样，测试片剂硬度。称重，考察平均片重。重新调节片重、压力以及出片。在用电动机启动压片机之前，必须调节好机器，消除压片的问题。

⑥启动机器电动机。检查产品的外观、片重、崩解度和硬度。依据规定，调节机器的压力、以使产品符合要求。

⑦撤除并用纱布清洁模具。

4．片剂包衣方法

糖衣和薄膜衣是最常见的包衣。与包糖衣相比，薄膜包衣具有操作简便、衣层薄、物料标准化、质量稳定、易于崩解、易于控制释放等优点。

片剂的包衣方法有多种，滚转包衣法是最普通的包衣方法。该法使用包衣锅，将片芯和衣料在锅中旋转中，形成包衣片。这种包衣法广泛用于医药、营养和食品工业的片剂、丸剂包衣。包衣锅一般是由不锈钢或铜制成；主要设备包括一个圆锥型包衣锅、动力传动装置、加热器，以及冷热鼓风设备、吸尘和吸湿气的真空装置等。包衣锅还可配备手动或自动的喷雾设备。可用于糖浆、混悬液或有机溶液的包衣。如果用有机溶液包衣，必须用防火包衣锅，配有鼓风和真空装置。

5．片剂的检查

（1）脆碎度　2000 版《中国药典》（一部）没有规定脆碎度和硬度的检查方法，由生产者自行控制。《中国药典》二部规定非包衣片应符合片剂脆碎度检查的要求。

脆碎度的检查方法如下：

本法用于检查非包衣片的脆碎情况及其他物理强度，如压碎强度等。

装置　内径约为286mm，深度为39mm，内壁抛光，一边可打开的透明耐磨塑料圆筒，筒内有一自中心向外壁延伸的弧形隔片（内径为80mm±1mm），使圆筒转动时，片剂产生滚动。圆筒直立固定于水平转轴上，转轴与电动机相连，转速为每分钟25转±1转。每转动一圈，片剂滚动或滑动至筒壁或其他片剂上。

检查法　片重为0.65g或以下者取若干片，使其总重约为6.5g；片重大于0.65g者取10片。用吹风机吹去脱落的粉末，精密称重，置圆筒中，转动100次。取出，同法除去粉末，精密称重，减失重量不得过1%，且不得检出断裂、龟裂及粉碎的片。本试验一般仅作1次。如减失重量超过1%时，可复检2次，3次的平均减失重量不得过1%，并不得检出断裂、龟裂及粉碎的片。

如供试品的形状或大小使片剂在圆筒中形成不规则滚动时，可调节圆筒的底座，使与桌面成约10°的角，试验时片剂不再聚集，能顺利下落。

对泡腾片及口嚼片等易吸水的制剂，操作时应注意防止吸湿（通常控制相对湿度小于40%）。

（2）片重差异　片剂的重量差异限度应符合下表之规定。抽取20片样品，精密称定总重量，并求得平均片重后，再分别精密称定片剂平均重量各药片的重量，每片重量与平均片重相比较（凡有标示片重的片剂，每片重量应与标示片重相比较），超出重量差异限度的药片不得多于2片，并不得有1片超出重量差异限度的一倍。

片剂重量差异限度表

片剂平均重量	重量差异限度
0.3g以下	+7.5%
0.3g或0.3g以上	+5.0%

（3）崩解时限

①将吊篮通过上端的不锈钢轴悬挂于金属支架上，浸入1000ml烧杯中，烧杯盛有温度在37±1℃的水，调节水位高度使吊篮上升时筛网在水面下25mm处，下降时筛网距烧杯底部25mm，支架上下移动的距离为55±2mm，往返速度为每分钟30~32次。

②除另有规定外，取药片6片，分别置上述吊篮的玻璃管中，每管各加1片，按上述方法检查，各片均应在15分钟内全部溶或崩解成碎粒，并通过筛网。如残存有小颗粒不能全部通过筛网时，应另取6片复试并在每管加入药片后随即加入挡板各1块，依法，均应符合规定。

③按上述方法检查糖衣片、浸膏片、半浸膏片或薄膜衣片的崩解时限，按上述方法检查，应在1小时内全部溶解崩解并通过筛网；全粉片应在30分钟内全部崩解。薄膜衣片可在盐酸溶液（9→1000）中进行检查。如残存有小颗粒不能全部通过筛网，就取6片各加挡板1块进行复试，均应符合定论。

凡规定检查溶出度的片剂，可不进行崩解时限检查含片、咀嚼片不检查崩解时限。

实验　芦丁片的制备

芦丁片[2] tabellae rutini 为《中华人民共和国卫生部药品标准》收载的制剂。本品含芦丁（$C_{27}H_{30}O_{16}\cdot 3H_2O$），应为标示量的 90.0～110.0%。芦丁由中药槐花米（Flos sophorae，槐 *Sophora japonica* 的干燥花和花蕾）中提取制得。

性状：本品为黄色或黄绿色片。

作用与用途：具有降低毛细血管的异常通透性和脆性的作用。主要用于防治高血压病的辅助治疗。

用法与用量：口服，一次 20～40mg，一日 60～120mg。

规格：20mg。

贮藏：遮光，密闭保存。

【实验材料】

仪器：混合机、磨粉机、筛（80 目、18 目、16 目）、普通天平、烘箱、单冲压片机、片剂硬度测定仪、片剂脆碎度测定仪、片剂崩解度测定仪、冲头（12mm、9mm）等。

药品和试剂：芦丁、淀粉、糊精、硬脂酸镁、乙醇等。

1．处方

芦丁	208g
淀粉	300g
糊精	100g
乙醇（60%）	300g
硬脂酸镁	66g

共制 1000 片

（每组学生可取十分之一量实验）

2．制法

将芦丁与淀粉按 4∶5 投入混合机中，干混 5min，然后在万能磨粉机内粉碎二遍，过 80 目筛。在细粉中加入剩余的淀粉、糊精，干混均匀，用 60% 乙醇制成适宜的软材。将软材挤压过 18 筛制粒。在 60～70℃干燥颗粒，控制含水量在 2%～5%。在干颗粒中加入硬脂酸镁，用 16 目钢丝筛整粒，混匀，压片，即得。

3．鉴别和含量测定

应符合芦丁片的国家药品标准。

4．检查

照片剂检查项下有关的各项规定检查芦丁片的片重差异、崩解时限和脆碎度。用一种硬度测定仪考察片剂硬度。

实验　元胡止痛片

元胡止痛片[3]（Yuanhu Zhitong Pian，Yuanhu Zhitong Tablets ）为《中华人民共和国药

典》收载的制剂。本品为半浸膏片，含香豆素类和生物碱化合物。

性状：本品为糖衣片或薄膜衣片，除去包衣后，显棕褐色；气香，味苦。

功能与主治：理气，活血，止痛。用于气滞血瘀的胃痛，胁痛，头痛及痛经等。

用法与用量：口服，一次 4～6 片，一日 3 次，或遵医嘱。

贮藏：密封。

【实验材料】

仪器：混合机、磨粉机、筛（100 目、20 目、18 目）、普通天平、烘箱、单冲压片机、包衣锅、喷枪、片剂硬度测定仪、片剂脆碎度测定仪、片剂崩解度测定仪等。

药品和试剂：延胡索（醋制）、白芷、Ⅳ号聚丙烯酸树脂、聚乙二醇 6000、滑石粉、钛白粉、硬脂酸镁、乙醇等。

1．处方

延胡索（醋制）	445g
白芷	223g
辅料	适量
制成薄膜包衣片	1000 片

（每组学生可取十分之一量实验）

2．制法：

（1）取经过灭菌的白芷 16.6g，粉碎成细粉（100 目）。

（2）剩余的白芷与延胡索粉碎成粗粉，用四倍量的 60% 乙醇浸泡 24 小时，加热回流 3 小时，收集提取液，再加三倍量的 60% 乙醇加热回流 2 小时，收集提取液，合并提取液，滤过，滤液浓缩成稠浸膏状。

（3）将上稠浸膏状加入上述细粉，制软材，过 20 目筛制粒，在 60～70℃干燥颗粒。过 18 目筛整粒，加硬脂酸镁 1%，混匀，压制成 100 片素片。

（4）包薄膜衣

①包衣料参考配方[4]

Ⅳ号聚丙烯酸树脂	6g
0.5%乙醇	200ml
聚乙二醇	6000 1.5 g
滑石粉	2.5g
钛白粉	2.5g
色素	适量

②操作　将滑石粉和钛白粉混匀，过 60 目筛，与其他包衣成分混匀，经胶体磨研磨后，制成包衣液。

③将素片置于包衣锅内加热风、翻动、预热 5 min，开动包衣锅，用喷枪喷包衣液。

④控制喷枪流和气流预热温度，以形成包衣，但片子不黏连为度。

3．鉴别

参见《中国药典》。

4．检查

按照片剂有关各项规定，检查片剂的外观、崩解时限、脆碎度和片重差异。

【思考题】

1．压片机的压力如何影响片剂的硬度？

2．崩解时间快，是否意味着生物利用度高？

3．存在这种可能：满足中国药典对片重差异的要求，但是未达到含量均一性要求。为什么？

4．生产者控制片剂硬度以保证片剂的特性，由片剂硬度反映的这些特性是什么？

5．为什么要包衣？

6．包糖衣和包薄膜衣有何不同？

7．何种薄膜衣料配方适合元胡止痛片的包衣？

参 考 文 献

1．国家药典委员会．中华人民共和国药典 一部，北京：化学工业出版社，2000，附录7

2．中华人民共和国卫生部．中华人民共和国卫生部药品标准－中药成方制剂十七分册．1998，257

3．中国国家药典委员会．中华人民共和国药典 一部，北京：化学工业出版社．2000，384

4．庄越，等．实用药物制剂技术．北京：人民卫生出版社．1999．P125～159

Exercise 9 Tablets

Exercise objectives

1. Practice and learn the general process to produce tablets.
2. Understand and learn the quality control of tablets.
3. Learn the basic requirement for tablet presses and the basic elements.

Instruction

Tablets[1-2] are solid preparations of various laminal shapes, usually round, and obtained by compressing uniform volumes of particles containing one or more active ingredients with suitable excipients. Tablets of traditional Chinese medicine are made of extracts of crude drugs, extracts of crude drugs with finely powdered crude drugs, or finely powdered crude drugs with suitable excipients. They may be classed as extract tablets, part - extract tablets and powdered crude drug tablets.

They are mainly conventional oral tablets, or lozenges, sublingual tablets, patches, chewable tablets, dispersible tablets, effervescent tablets, vaginal tablets, and extended release or controlled release tablets, enteric coated tablets etc.

Compressed tablets are manufactured by either wet granulation method or by dry granulation method or by direct compression. Except for the drug substances that are volatile, thermolabile and unstable on exposure to moisture, most of drug substances can be made into tablets by wet granulation.

1. General requirement for preparation of tablets

(1) The medicaments should be mixed with the excipients thoroughly. Tablets containing medicaments toxic or potent in nature or those administered in small dosage are dispersed uniformly in a way appropriate for the substance concerned.

(2) Tablets containing volatile or thermolabile substances are processed in a way to avoid loss on heating. The moisture content of the granules used in the process should be controlled to meet the requirement of processing and to prevent deliquescence, mold contamination, deterioration or loss of effectiveness during storage.

(3) Tablets containing drug substances with unpleasant odour, taste or irritating properties, or unstable on exposure to moisture or light, may be coated with sugar or film. Tablets are enteric coated when the drug substance can be destroyed by gastric fluid or when it is to be released in the intestine. Vaginal tablets are made for topical use in vagina. Effervescent tablets, buccal tablets, chewable tablets etc. are made for some drugs that are

needed.

(4) Tables have a clean, smooth and uniformly coloured surface without breakage; they are sufficiently hard to withstand handling without cracking.

(5) Generally, tablets should be preserved in tightly closed containers.

2. The general steps involved in a wet granulation process

(1) The powdered ingredients are weighed and mixed carefully. Tablets containing medicaments toxic in nature or those administered in small doses are dispersed uniformly in a way appropriate for the substances concerned.

(2) The granulation solution (wetter or binder) is prepared.

(3) The powders and the granulation solution are kneaded to proper consistency, forming a lump when holding and breaking up when pressing softly.

(4) The wet mass is forced through a screen or wet granulator.

(5) The granules are dried in an oven or a fluidized bed dryer at the proper temperature that is chosen according to the characteristic of the medicaments. The moisture content of the granules used in the process should be controlled to meet the requirement of the processing and to prevent deliquescence, mold contamination, deterioration or loss of effectiveness during storage.

(6) The dried granules are screened to a suitable size for compression.

(7) A lubricant (and a disintegrating agent) is mixed with the granule. Volatile medicaments may be added in different ways: spraying a solution of the drug onto granules, or by encapsulation, or by inclusion with cyclodextrine.

(8) The qualified granules are compressed into the finished tablet.

3. Tablet press

The tablet press is the main equipment for production of tablets. Rotary tablet presses and high speed rotary tablet presses become the main products with high capacity and good quality. The advanced High Speed Rotary Tablet Presses are full closed and use stainless steel so as to ensure clean inside and to completely divide from outside, having auto control system of ejection of unqualified tablet. A powder suction unit is attached to take in the residual, it can absorb the powder during the operation. The capacity is more than 200,000 tablets/hr.

Single punch tablet presses are commonly used in the pharmaceutics laboratory.

(1) TDP Single punch tablet press

The machine is designed for pressing round tablets from various granular materials, applicable in a lab used for research and development and for small - scale production. As its feature, it is a small desk - top continuous press driven by motor or man - power. Only one set of punch and die is mounted. The depth of the filling material and the thickness of the tablets can be adjusted.

Max. Pressure: 1.5 kn; Max. diameter of tablet: 12 mm; Max. depth of fill: 11mm

Max. Thickness of Tablet 6 mm; Capacity: 6000 tablets/h

(2) ZDY8 Heavy – Duty Single – Punch Tablet Press

It is a heavy duty single tablet press designed to produce larger tablets, which is used in pharmaceutical laboratory, nutraceutical companies, the chemical and other related industries. It is great for small – batch production.

This machine can press special – shaped, ring – like tablets of different kinds, and can also press tablets both sides are impressed trademarks, letters and simple patterns.

Max. capacity: 90 tablets/min; Max. diameter of tablet: 18mm; Max. depth of filling: 20mm; Max. Pressure: 80kn.

Notice for Setting up and operating Single punch tablet press:

①Install the lower – punch in machine and adjust tablet – weight regulator.

②Fix the die on the plate and adjust tablet – release regulator.

③Install upper – punch and adjust pressure regulator, making the upper – punch going into the cavity in the middle of the die, using the handwheel.

④Scoop ingredients into feeding – boot and hopper. Turn the wheel by hand to try compressing tablets and collects samples of product.

⑤Break sample tablets between fingers to test hardness. Weigh samples of tablets to verify average weight. Adjusts machine controls again to eliminate tablet defects before starting machine by motor.

⑥Start the motor of the machine. Examine tablet weighs, and test samples for hardness, disintegration and defects, such as surface chips and pits, excessive brittleness, using scale, and hardness tester; to verify machine setup. Route sample to lab for analysis, according to procedure. Adjusts machine pressure and tension to remove product flaws and ensure conformity to product specifications. Records product information.

⑦Removes and cleans dies, using swabs.

4. Method of coating

Sugar coating system and film coating system are most commonly applied to tablets. Over the sugar coating the film coating has advantages of improving productivity, thinner coats, standardizing materials, more stable quality, easier disintegration, and easier control of release.

Several methods are used for tablet coating. The most popular coating method utilizes a roll coating pan for rolling core tablets with coat materials to form coated tablets. It is widely used in the pharmaceutical, nutritional and food industries for coating tablets or pills. Pans may be made of stainless steel or copper. The operating mechanism is mounted on conical rollers. They are available with a gear motor and a heater, and may be fitted with cold or hot air individual blowers as well as a vacuum device to extract dust and moisturized air reducing drying time in the process. These coating pans may also be equipped with manual or automatic spraying devices. They may be used to coat with syrup, solids in suspension or organic solvents. If a flammable coating solution is used, flameproof pans must be fitted with air blowers and vacuum devices.

5. Tests

(1) Friability and hardness The uncoated tablets should comply with the test for tablet friability, described in the Pharmacopoeia of People's Republic of China (2000). The hardness of tablets may be tested to control the quality by manufacturers.

The following provides guidelines for the friability determination of compressed, uncoated tablets. The test procedure presented in this chapter is generally applicable to most compressed tablets, and supplements other physical strength measurements, such as tablet crushing strength.

Apparatus Use a 286 mm (i.d.) drum, about 39 mm in depth, of transparent synthetic polymer with polished internal surfaces, and not subject to static build – up (see Fig.). One side of the drum is removable. The tablets are tumbled at each turn of the drum by a curved projection that extends from the middle of the drum to the outer wall. The drum is attached to the horizontal axis of a device that rotates at approximately 25 ± 1 rpm. Thus, at each turn the tablets roll or slide and fall onto the drum wall or onto each other.

Procedure For tablets weighing up to 650 mg each, use a 6.5g sample. For tablets weighing over 650 mg each, a 10 – tablet sample is sufficient. Place the tablets on a No. 10 sieve and remove any loose dust with the aid of air pressure or a soft brush. Accurately weigh the tablet sample, and place the tablets in the drum. Rotate the drum 100 times, and remove the tablets. Remove any loose dust from the tablets as before and weigh.

Generally, the test is run once. If the results are doubtful or if the weight loss is greater than 1%, the test should be repeated twice and the mean of the three tests determined. A maximum weight loss of not more than 1% of the weight of the tablets being tested is considered acceptable and any tablets broken, chapped and smashed are not picked up. If tablet size or shape causes irregular tumbling, adjust the drum so that its axis forms a 10° angle with the base and the tablets no longer bind together when lying next to each other, which prevents them from falling freely.

In the cases of effervescent tablets, chewable tablets and hydroscopic tablets, care must be taken to perform the test quickly enough to prevent moisture absorption (relative humidity is not more than 40%).

(2) Weight variation Tablets should comply with the following requirements stated in the table below.

Average weight	Weight variation limit
Less than 0.3g	± 7.5%
0.3g or more	± 5%

Procedure Weigh accurately 20 tablets and calculate the average weight, then weigh individually each of the 20 tablets. Compare the weight of each tablet with the labelled tablet weight (if no labelled weight is stated, compare the weight of each tablet with the average weight calculated). Not more than 2 of the individual weights exceed the weight variation limit stated in the table above and none doubles the limit.

Sugar, film and enteric coated tablets should be tested before coating to show that the tablet cores comply with the above requirements. Tablets need not be tested again after coating.

(3) Disintegration test Carry out the test as described under the disintegration test as follows. Unless otherwise specified, all the tablets should comply with the specified requirements. Where a dissolution test is prescribed, a disintegration test may not be required. A disintegration test is not required for sublingual tablets or chewable tablets.

①Apparatus The apparatus mainly consists of a basket – rack assembly with disk and a motion device for raising and lowing the basket in the liquid medium at a constant rate between 30 ~ 32 cycles per minute through a distance of 55 mm ± 2mm (see Fig.2).

②Procedure The basket is suspended in a 1000 ml beaker, maintained at 37℃ ± 1℃, the volume of the fluid in the vessel is adjusted appropriately so that at the highest point of the upward stroke the wire mesh remains at least 25 mm below the surface of the fluid and descends to a distance not less than 25 mm from the bottom of the vessel on downward stroke. Unless specified otherwise, place 1 tablet in each of the 6 tubes of the basket, add a disk and operate the apparatus. Tablets of powdered crude drugs disintegrate completely within 30 minutes; tablets of extracts (part – extracts), sugar – coating tablets disintegrate completely within 1 hours; common tablets disintegrate completely within 15 minutes. If 1 tablet fails to disintegrate completely, repeat the operation with another 6 tablets. All the tablets should comply with the test.

TABELLAE RUTINI

Rutin tablet[3] is a preparation recorded in the Pharmaceutics Standards of Health Ministry of the People's Republic of China. It contains rutin ($C_{27}H_{30}O_{16} \cdot 3H_2O$) that is 90.0% ~ 110.0% of labelled weight. Rutin is extracted from Flos sophorae.

Description Yellow, or yellowish green tablets.

Action and Indications To increase the strength of the capillaries (blood vessels) and to decrease their extraordinary permeability. It is mainly applied to auxiliary prevention and cure of hypertension.

Usage and dosage oral, 20 ~ 40mg. 60 ~ 120mg a day.

Specification 20 mg.

Storage Protected from light, store sealed.

Exercise materials

Instruments: Mixer, mill, screens (80, 18, 16 mesh), scale, oven, single punch tablet press, tablets hardness testing Instrument, tablet friability tester, tablet disintegration tester and punches (12, 9 mm), etc.

Drugs and reagents: Rutin, starch, dextrin, magnesium stearate, ethanol etc.

Methods

1. Formulation

Rutin	208g
Starch	300g
Dextrin	100g
Ethanol 60%	300g
magnesium stearate	66g

Made into 1000 tablets.

(the tenth for student's exercise)

2. Procedure

Mix rutin and starch (4:5) in a mixer for 5 min. The mixture is pulverized in a mill twice, and pass through 80 mesh screens. Add remainder starch and dextrin to the screened powder, and mix well. Knead the mixture to wet mass with 60% ethanol. Force the mass through 18 mesh screen to granulate. Dry the granules at 60 ~ 70℃, making the water content being 2 ~ 5%. Add magnesium stearate to the dried granules. The mixed granules are screened to 16 mesh. Compress the qualified granules into tablets with a single punch tablet press.

3. Identification and Assay

Comply with the national drug standard for rutin tablets.

4. Test

Test weight variation, disintegration and friability for rutin tablets, according to the specifications under the tablet tests. Test hardness for rutin tablets, using a hardness testing instrument.

Yuanhu Zhitong Pian

Yuanhu Zhitong tablets[4] is a preparation recorded in the Pharmacopoeia of People's Republic of China.

The tablet is made of Rhizoma Corydalis and Radix Angelicae Dahuricae. It is a part-extract tablet, containing alkaloids and coumarins.

Description Sugar or film coated tablets, with brown core; odour, aromatic; taste, bitter.

Action To regulate the flow of qi, promote blood circulation and relieve pain.

Indications Gastralgia, hypochondriac pain, headache or dysmellorrhea due to stagnation of qi and blood.

Usage and dosage 4 ~ 6 tablets, 3 times a day, or follow the physician's advice.

Storage Preserve in tightly closed containers.

Exercise materials

Instruments: Mixer, mill, sieves (100, 20, 18, mesh), scale, oven, single punch tablet press, coating pan, spray gun, tablets hardness testing Instrument, tablet friability tester, tablet disintegration tester and punches, etc.

Drugs and reagents: Rhizoma Corydalis, Radix Angelicae Dahuricae, magnesium stearate, ethanol, polypropylene resin (Ⅳ), polyethylene Glycol 6000, talc, titanium oxide, etc.

Exercise Method

1. Formulation

Rhizoma Corydalis (processed with vinegar)	445g
Radix Angelicae Dahuricae	223g
Excipients available amount	
Made into 1000 film-coating tablets	
(the tenth for student' Exercise)	

2. Procedure

(1) Pulverize 16.6 g of sterilized Radix Angelicae Dahuricae to fine powder, and screen the powder through 100 mesh.

(2) Pulverize the remains of Radix Angelicae Dahuricae and Rhizoma Corydalis to coarse powder. Macerate the coarse powder with 4 times volume of 60% ethanol for 24 hours, heat under reflux for 3 hours and collect the extract. To the residue add 3 times volume of 60% ethanol, heat under reflux again for 2 hours and collect the extract. Combine

the extracts and filter. Concentrate the filtrate to a thick extract (relative density 1.2).

(3) Add the above fine powder, make wet mass. Force the mass through 20 mesh screen to granulate. Dry the granules at 60 ~ 70℃. Add 1% of magnesium stearate to the dried granules. The mixed granules are screened to 18 mesh. Compress the qualified granules into tablets with a single punch tablet press.

(4) Film coating

① Coating materials[5]

Polypropylene resin (Ⅳ)	6g
0.5% ethanol	200ml
Polyethylene Glycol 6000	1.5g
Talc	2.5g
Titanium oxide	2.5g
Pigment	

② Mix talc and titanium oxide, screen the mixture through 60 mesh. Mix the powder with other ingredients and mill the mixture in a colloid mill to form a coating suspension.

③ Core (uncoated) tablets are placed and agitated inside the coating pan while the coating pan is blown with hot air for 5 min, rotated at a selected speed to provide movement of the tablets. A spray gun is used to deliver coating suspension.

④ Airflow pre – heated to the desired temperature and controlled at the desired flow rate is applied to the tablets. The evaporation of coating solvent (s) forms the film or layer around the tablets without sticking to each other.

3. Identification

Refer to the Pharmacopoeia of People's Republic of China.

4. Test

Test weight variation, disintegration and friability for rutin tablets, according to the specifications under the tablet tests. Test hardness for rutin tablets, using a hardness testing instrument.

Questions

1. How does compaction pressure of tablet press influence tablet hardness?

2. When a tablet has a rapid disintegration time, it will always have a large bioavailability. Is that right?

3. It is possible for tablets to pass the PPRC weight variation requirement but fail the content uniformity requirement. How is this possible?

4. Manufacturers monitor tablet hardness to ensure certain characteristics in their tablets. What are desired characteristics measured by tablet hardness?

5. Why do we coat tablets ?

6. What are the differences between sugar coating and film coating?

7. Which formulation of coating materials for Yuanhu Zhitong tablets is the best?

References

1. Pharmacopoeia Commission of PRC. Pharmacopoeia of P.R. of China. Volume I. Beijing: Chemical Industry Press. 2000, Appendix 7

2. Pharmacopoeia Commission of PRC. Pharmacopoeia of P.R. of China (English edition). Volume I. Beijing: Chemical Industry Press. 1997, Appendix I A – 6

3. Health Ministry of P.R. of China. Pharmaceutical Standards of Health Ministry of P.R. of China – Preparations of TCM Vol. 17. 1998, 257

4. Pharmacopoeia Commission of PRC. Pharmacopoeia of P.R. of China. Volume I. Beijing: Chemical Industry Press. 2000, 384

5. Zhuang Yue, etc. Practical Skills of Pharmaceutical Preparation. Beijing: People's Health Press. 1999. P125 ~ 159

实验十　胶　囊　剂

【实验目的】

1. 通过学习和实验，掌握胶囊剂的制备方法与质量控制要求。

2. 熟悉胶囊剂崩解时限和内容物流动性的测定方法及其意义。

【实验指导】

胶囊剂[1-2]是用具一定形状和不同装量的硬质囊壳或软质囊材制成的固体制剂，通常为口服给药。其内容物可以是固体、液体或糊状体，其中含有一种或多种活性成分，需要时可以加入适量的赋形剂，如溶剂、稀释剂、润滑剂和崩解剂等。中药胶囊剂可分为硬胶囊剂、软胶囊剂和肠溶胶囊剂三类。

硬胶囊剂　硬胶囊剂系指将药材提取物或药材粉末加辅料制成均匀粉末、颗粒、小丸、半固体或液体，充填于空心胶囊而制成。空心胶囊由囊帽和囊体两部分组成。一般将药物充填于囊体，再将囊帽套合其上，封口即得。

软胶囊剂　软胶囊剂系指将一定量的药材提取物加适宜的辅料密封于球形、椭圆形或其他形状的软质囊材中制备而成。软质囊材可由明胶、甘油和/或其他适宜的药用材料制成，比硬质囊壳厚。其内容物一般以液体形式通过滴制法或压制法制成软胶囊。

肠溶胶囊剂　肠溶胶囊剂系指将硬胶囊或软胶囊经药用高分子材料处理或用其他适宜方法加工而成。也可将药物粉末或颗粒包肠溶衣，再充填于普通胶囊中而制得。肠溶胶囊剂是一种控释制剂，它不溶于胃液，但能在肠液中释放活性成分。

1. 胶囊剂生产和贮存的一般要求

(1) 胶囊内容物不引起囊壳的变形和变质，但囊壳能在消化液中崩解，释放有效成分。

(2) 小剂量药物，应先用适宜的稀释剂稀释，并混合均匀。

(3) 胶囊剂应外观整洁、光滑，不得有黏结、变形或破裂现象，并无异臭。

(4) 胶囊剂一般应密封贮存于不超过30℃的环境中。

2. 微粒的测定

硬胶囊内容物通常是固体粉末或颗粒，其可压性和流动性能影响胶囊的填充和装量的准确性。采用下列方法测定内容物的微粒特性。

(1) 可压性　取胶囊内容物10g，慢慢倾入25ml刻度量筒中，轻轻敲拍量筒壁，直至内容物体积不再变化为止。分别以内容物重量除以其敲拍前后的体积，计算得初始松密度ρ_b（g/cm^3）和压缩松密度ρ_p（g/cm^3）。由下列公式算得压缩百分比：

$$压缩百分比 = 100（\rho_p - \rho_b）/\rho p$$

(2) 休止角　休止角可采用固定漏斗法测量。试验时，取漏斗1个，使其下缘距水平面8cm高，然后使胶囊内容物10g通过该漏斗，样品在水平面上形成粒堆，粒堆斜边与水平面之间的夹角即为休止角。

（3）均匀性系数　均匀性系数由 10g 内容物样品筛分而得。振荡筛配备有八个标准筛子，筛孔从 0.075 到 1.7mm 不等，试验时以 80 次/分的速度振荡 120 秒。通过 60% 样品的筛孔尺寸除以通过 10%样品的筛孔尺寸所得的数值就是均匀性系数。

3．检查

（1）崩解时限

照《中国药典》一部附录规定的方法，在 37℃水浴中用升降式崩解仪测定该胶囊剂的崩解时限。硬胶囊剂应在 30 分钟内、软胶囊应在 1 小时内全部崩解并通过筛网（囊壳碎片除外）。

（2）水分测定

照《中国药典》一部附录规定的方法，测定该胶囊剂内容物的水分含量。除另有规定外，硬胶囊剂固体内容物水分含量不得超过 9.0%。

（3）装量差异

照《中国药典》一部附录规定的方法检查，胶囊剂每粒装量与标识装量相比较，应在 ±10.0% 以内。

实验　独一味胶囊

独一味胶囊（Duyiwei Jiaonang）收载于《中华人民共和国药典》，是由独一味提取加工制成的胶囊剂[3-4]。独一味[5]，藏药名为达巴，为 *Lamiophlomis rotata*（Benth.）Kudo. 的干燥全草，含有黄酮类等水溶性活性成分。独一味胶囊每粒含木犀草素（$C_{15}H_{10}O_6$），不得少于 0.80mg。

性状：本品为胶囊剂，内容物为深棕色的颗粒或粉末；味微苦。

功能和主治：活血止痛，化瘀止血。用于多种外科手术后的刀口疼痛、出血，外伤骨折，筋骨扭伤，风湿痹痛以及崩漏、痛经、牙龈肿痛、出血等。

用法和用量：口服，一次 3 粒，一日 3 次，7 天为一疗程；或必要时服用。

注意：孕妇慎用。

规格：每粒装 0.3g。

贮藏：密封。

【实验材料】

仪器：胶囊充填机，烧瓶（1000ml，500ml），容量瓶，25 ml 刻度量筒，漏斗，加热器，真空过滤瓶，布氏漏斗（Φ9cm），天平，水浴，研钵，筛子，半圆式量角器，不锈钢刮刀，烘箱，层析缸，薄层板（硅胶 G），离心分离机，崩解度测试仪，紫外线－可见分光光度计等。

药品和试剂：独一味药材，淀粉，空心胶囊，芦丁，乙醇，甲醇，氯仿，亚硝酸钠，硝酸铝，磷钼酸。

【实验方法】

1．处方

独一味　　1000g

淀粉　　适量

全方制成　　1000 粒胶囊

（学生实验可用五十分之一量）

2．制法

（1）粉碎和煎煮　取独一味药材，粉碎，加适量水煎煮 3 次，每次 1 小时，合并煎液，滤过。

（2）浓缩与干燥　取滤过液，浓缩成相对密度为 1.30 的清膏，在 80℃以下干燥，并粉碎成细粉。

（3）制粒　提取物细粉，加适量淀粉，制成颗粒，干燥。

（4）填充　药物颗粒装入胶囊，即得。

3．鉴别与含量测定

（1）鉴别　取本品内容物 0.3g，加乙醇 5ml，加热回流 10 分钟，滤过，取滤液 2ml，浓缩至约 1ml，作为供试品溶液。另取独一味对照药材 1g，同法制成对照药材溶液。照薄层色谱法（中国药典 2000 年版一部附录）试验，吸取上述两种溶液各 5μl，分别点于同一硅胶 G 薄层板上（不活化），以氯仿－甲醇（4∶1）为展开剂，展开，取出，晾干，喷以磷钼酸 105°C 加热约 15 分钟。供试品色谱中，在与对照药材色谱相应的位置上，显相同颜色的斑点。

（2）含量测定

对照品溶液的制备　精密称取在 120℃减压干燥至恒重的芦丁对照品 200mg，置 100ml 量瓶中，加 70%乙醇 70ml，置水浴上微热使溶解，放冷，加 70%乙醇至刻度，摇匀。精密量取 10ml，置 100ml 量瓶中，加水至刻度，摇匀，即得（每 1ml 中含无水芦丁 0.2mg）。

标准曲线的制备　精密量取对照品溶液 1.0、2.0、3.0、4.0、5.0、6.0ml，分别置 25ml 量瓶中，加水至 6ml，加 5%亚硝酸钠溶液 1ml，混匀，放置 6 分钟，加 10%硝酸铝溶液 1ml，摇匀，放置 6 分钟，加氢氧化钠试液 10ml，再加水至刻度，摇匀，放置 15 分钟；以相应的溶液为空白。照分光光度法（《中国药典》附录），在 500nm 波长处测定吸收度，以吸收度为纵坐标、浓度为横坐标，绘制标准曲线。

测定法　取本品 20 粒的内容物，精密称定，研细，取 0.6g，精密称定，置 100ml 量瓶中，加 70%乙醇 70ml，置水浴上微热并时时振摇 30 分钟，放冷，加 70%乙醇至刻度，摇匀，3000rpm 离心 20 分钟，精密量取上清液 1ml，置 25ml 量瓶中，照标准曲线的制备项下的方法，自“加水至 6ml”起，依法测定吸收度，从标准曲线上读出供试品溶液中芦丁的重量，计算，即得。每粒胶囊不得少于 20.0mg 芦丁。木犀草素的含量测定采用高效液相色谱法。

实验　补肾强身胶囊

补肾强身胶囊[6]（Bushen Qiangshen Jiaonang）是卫生部药品标准收载的中药制剂。本品由五味中药的复方制成，其中淫羊藿为小檗科植物淫羊藿 *Epimedium brevicornum* Maxim.、箭叶淫羊藿 *Epimedium sagittatum*（Sieb.et Zucc.）Maxim.、柔毛淫羊藿 *Epimedium pubescens* Maxim.、巫山淫羊藿 *Epimedium wushanense* T.S.Ying、或朝鲜淫羊藿 *Epimedium koreanum* Nakai 的干燥地上部分，含淫羊藿苷（icariin）等黄酮类化合物。金樱子为蔷薇科植物金樱子 *Rosa laevigata* Michx. 的干燥成熟果实。菟丝子为旋花科植物菟丝子 *Cuscuta chinensis* Lam. 的干燥成熟种子。女贞子为木犀科植物女贞 *Ligustrum lucidum* Ait. 的干燥成熟果实含齐墩果酸（Oleanolic acid）、熊果酸（Ursolic acid）等三萜类化合物。狗脊为蚌壳蕨科植物金毛狗脊 *Cibotium barometz*（L.）J.Sm. 的干燥根茎。

性状：本品为胶囊剂，内容物为棕色至棕褐色的粉末；味微酸。

功能与主治：补肾强身。用于腰酸足软，头晕耳鸣，眼花心悸，阳痿遗精。

用法与用量：口服，一次 3 粒，一日 3 次。

规格：每粒装 0.3g。

贮藏：密封。

【实验材料】

仪器：烧杯（1000ml，500ml）、电炉、抽滤器、水浴、不锈钢盘、真空干燥箱、研钵、药筛、胶囊填充器、天平、崩解测定仪。

药品和试剂：淫羊藿、金樱子、菟丝子、女贞子（制）、狗脊（制）和空胶囊。

【实验方法】

1．处方

淫羊藿	225g
金樱子	135g
菟丝子	135g
女贞子（制）	135g
狗脊（制）	135g

2．制法

（1）煎煮：取淫羊藿、金樱子、菟丝子饮片加适量水煎煮二次，第一次 2 小时，第二次 1.5 小时，合并煎液，滤过，静置 8～12 小时；

（2）粉碎：取女贞子（制）、狗脊（制）粉碎成细粉，过六号筛；

（3）浓缩：取滤出的上清液，浓缩为相对密度为 1.16～1.18（70～80℃）的清膏；

（4）制粒和装胶囊：将药粉加入清膏，拌匀，在 80℃以下干燥，粉碎，过五号筛，装入胶囊，即得。

3．检查

应符合胶囊剂有关的各项规定。

4．计算

计算提取淫羊藿、金樱子和菟丝子的提取率、每粒胶囊的含量和胶囊的得率。

【思考题】

1．与其他剂型相比，胶囊剂在剂型上有哪些优点？

2．简述胶囊剂的制备方法和操作要点。

参 考 文 献

1．国家药典委员会．中华人民共和国药典 2000 年版（一部）．北京：化学工业出版社．2000，附录 11

2．The Stationary Office．British Pharmacopoeia（Volume II，2000 Edition）．London，2002，1655

3．国家药典委员会．中华人民共和国药典 2000 年版（增补本）．北京：化学工业出版社．2002，17

4．国家药典委员会．中华人民共和国药典 2000 年版（一部）．北京：化学工业出版社．2000，533

5．中华人民共和国卫生部．中华人民共和国卫生部药品标准，藏药，第一册，73

6．中华人民共和国卫生部．中华人民共和国卫生部药品标准，中药成方制剂，第 4 册，87

Exercise 10 Capsules

Learning Objectives

Following study of the capsules, the student should be able to:

1. Keep informed on preparation of capsules and grasp their requirements for control of the quality.

2. Be familiar with disintegration study and understand how to test the flowability of granules or powder.

Instruction

1. Introduction

Capsules[1-3] are solid preparations with hard or soft shells of a various shapes and capacities, usually intended for oral administration. The contents of capsules may be solid, liquid or of a paste-like consistency. They consist of one or more active ingredients with or without excipients such as solvents, diluents, lubricants and disintegrating agents. Three categories of capsules may be distinguished: hard capsules, soft capsules and gastro-resistant capsules.

Hard capsules Hard capsules have shells consisting of two prefabricated cylindrical sections one end of which is rounded and closed, the other being open. Crude drug extracts or crude drug powder with or without excipients, usually in uniform granules, powder, micro-pills, semi-solid, or liquid are filled into one of the sections which is then closed by slipping the other section over it.

Soft capsules Soft capsules have thicker shells than those of hard capsules. They are prepared by drip-feed or compression method. The medicament with proper excipients, usually prepared in liquid form, are filled and sealed in spherical, elliptical or other shaped soft capsules made of gelatin, glycerin and/or other suitable materials.

Gastro-resistant capsules Gastro-resistant capsules are modified release capsules that are intended to resist the gastric fluid and to release their active ingredients in the intestinal fluids. They are prepared by providing hard or soft capsules with a gastro-resistant shell (enteric capsules) or by filling capsules with granules or with particles covered with a gastro-resistant coating.

2. Requirements for production and storage of capsules

(1) The contents of capsules do not cause deformation and deterioration of shell. The shell, however, is attacked by the digestive fluids and the contents are released.

(2) Potent medicaments given in small doses are usually mixed thoroughly with a suitable diluents before filling.

(3) Capsules should have a clean, smooth surface and well shaped without adhesion, deformation or breakage. Capsules should not have strange odour.

(4) Capsules should be stored in well – closed container, at a temperature not exceeding 30℃, unless specified otherwise.

3. Characterization of particles

The contents of hard capsules are solid state powder or granules. Their micromeritic properties will affect the filling of the capsules.

(1) Compressibility Ten grams of the contents are poured lightly into a 25 ml graduated cylinder. The powder or the granules are tapped until no further change in volume observed. Powder bulk density, ρ_b ($g \cdot cm^{-3}$) and powder tapped density, ρ_p ($g \cdot cm^{-3}$) are calculated as the weight of the powder divided by its volume before and after tapping, respectively. Percentage compressibility is computed from the following equation:

$$\text{compressibility } \% = 100\ (\rho_p - \rho_b)\ /\rho p.$$

(2) Angle of repose Angle of repose is measured using a stationary funnel method for the heap of granules formed by passing 10 g of the sample through a funnel at a height of 8 cm from the horizontal surface.

(3) Uniformity coefficient Uniformity coefficient is obtained by sieve analysis of 10 g of the powdered material The sieve shaker is fitted with eight standard sieves ranging in size from 0.075 to 1.7 mm and vibrated at a setting of 80 for 120 s. Uniformity coefficient is measured as the numerical value arrived at by dividing the width of the sieve opening that will pass 60% of the sample by the width of sieve opening that will pass 10% of the sample.

4. Tests

(1) *Disintegration test*

Disintegration time is measured for three replicates using single basket disintegration testing system at 37℃ according to the Appendix of *Pharmacopoeia of P.R.China* (Vol.1). The hard capsules should disintegrate within 30 minutes and the soft capsules disintegrate and pass through the gauze within 1 hour.

(2) *Water determination*

The water content in the solid contents of this hard capsule, is determined by the loss on drying described in Determination of Water (Appendix, *Pharmacopoeia of P.R.China* (Vol.1). Unless otherwise specified, the water content of hard capsule is not more than 9.0%.

(3) Volume

The weight variation limit of 10 capsules should be within ±10.0%.

Duyiwei Capsules

Duyiwei Capsules (Duyiwei Jiaonang)[4] is a preparation included in the *Pharmacopoeia of People's Republic of China* (Vol.1).

Duyiwei Capsules are prepared with *Radix Lamiophlomidis Ratatae*, a Tibetan drug[5], which contains water – soluble active ingredients such as flavonoid. The content of luteolin ($C_{15}H_{10}O_6$) flavone per capsule is not less than 0.80 mg.

Description Capsules containing deep – brown granules or power. Taste, slightly bitter.

Action To activate blood circulation and alleviate pain, to remove *blood stasis* and arrest bleeding.

Indications Aching and bleeding after surgeries, traumatic injuries, strain of the bones and muscles, arthralgia due to *wind – dampness*, metrorrhagia, dysmenorrheal, painful swelling, of the gingival, bleeding, etc.

Usage and dosage 3 capsules, 3 times a day, 7 days for treatment, or taken when necessary.

Precaution Use with caution in pregnancy.

Specification 0.3g per capsule.

Storage Preserve in well – closed containers.

Exercise materials

Radix Lamiophlomidis Ratatae, starch, capsule vacuous, rutin, ethanol, methanol, chloroform, sodium nitrite, aluminum nitrate, phosphomolybdic acid, capsule filler, flasks (1000ml, 500ml), volumetric flask, 25 ml graduated cylinder, funnel, heater, vacuum filter, Buchner funnel (φ9cm), balance, water baths, mortar, sieves, protractor, steel spatula, oven, tanks, thin layer plates (silica gel G), centrifuge, single basket disintegration testing apparatus, UV – Visible spectrophotometer, etc.

Exercise Method

1. Formulation

Radix Lamiophlomidis Ratatae	1000g
Starch	Q. S.

(The quantity may be reduced for the student's exercise.)

2. Procedure

(1) Pulverization and Decoction Pulverize 1000g of *Radix Lamiophlomidis Ratatae*, decoct with an appropriate quantity of water for 3 times, each 1 hour. Combine the decoc-

tions and filter.

(2) Concentration and Drying Concentrate the filtrate to a liquid extract with a relative density of 1.30, and dry below 80℃.

(3) Granulating Add a quantity of starch to make granules, and make them dry.

(4) Packing Pack them to make 1000 capsules.

3. Identification and assay

(1) Identification To 0.3 g of the content, add 5 ml of ethanol, heat under reflux for 10 minutes, and filter. Concentrate 2 ml of filtrate to about 1 ml as the test solution. Prepare a solution with 1 g of Herba lamiophlomidis Rotatae reference drug as the reference drug solution in the same manner. Carry out the method for thin layer chromatography (Appendix, *Pharmacopoeia of P.R.China*), using silica gel G as the coating substance and a mixture of chloroform – methanol (4:1) as the mobile phase. Apply separately 5 μl of the two solutions to the plate (non – actived). After developing and removal of the plate, dry it in air, spray with phosphomolybdic acid, heat at 105°C for 15 minutes, the spots in the chromatogram obtained with the test solution correspond in position and colour to the spots in the chromatogram obtained with the reference solution.

(2) Assay *Standard preparation* Weigh accurately 200 mg of rutin, previously dried in vacuum to constant weight at 120℃, in a 100ml volumetric flask, add 70 ml of 70% ethanol and heat gently to dissolve on a water bath, cool and dilute with 70% ethanol to volume, and mix well. Transfer accurately 10 ml to a 100 ml volumetric flask, dilute to volume with water and mix well, used as the standard solution, containing 0.2 mg of anhydrous rutin per ml.

Preparation of calibration curve Measure accurately 1.0, 2.0, 3.0, 4.0, 5.0 and 6.0 ml of the standard solution in 25 ml volumetric flask separately, add water for each to 6 ml, and add 1 ml of 5% sodium nitrite solution, mix well, allow to stand for 6 minutes, then add 1 ml of a solution of 10% aluminum nitrate solution, mix well and allow to stand for 15 minutes. Carry out the method for spectrophotometry (Appendix, *Pharmacopoeia of P.R.China*), measure the absorbance at 500 nm, taking the reagent solution as a blank, plot calibration curve, using absorbance as ordinate and concentration as abscissa.

Procedure Grind the content of 20 capsules, weighed accurately, to fine powder, weigh accurately 0.6 g of the powder in a 100 ml volumetric flask, add 70 ml of ethanol, warm on a water bath for 30 minutes and shake constantly, cool and dilute to volume with 70% ethanol, centrifuge at the speed of 3000rpm for 20 minutes. Transfer accurately 1 ml of the supernatant to a 25 ml volumetric flask, carry out the procedure as the described under the preparation of the calibration curve, beginning at the words "add water for each to 6 ml", measure the absorbance, read out the weight of rutin in the test solution from the calibration curve, and calculate. The content of rutin per capsule is not less than 20.0mg. Assay of luteolin in the capsule is performed with HPLC method.

Bushen Qiangshen Capsules (Bushen Qiangshen Jiaonang)

Bushen Qiangshen Capsules, a tonic TCM preparation, has been marketed in China for many years. It is b ased on a multi – herb formula, in which Herba Epimedii originates from the dry aerial party of *Epimedium brevicornum* Maxim., *Epimedium sagittatum* (Sieb. et Zucc.) Maxim., *Epimedium pubescens* Maxim., *Epimedium wushanense* T. S. Ying, or *Epimedium koreanum* Nakai, containing flavonoids such as icariin; Frumctus Rosae Laevigatae is the dry mature fruits of *Rosa laevigata* Michx.; Semen Cuscutae is the dry mature seeds of *Cuscuta chinensis* Lam.; Fructus Ligustri Lucidi is the dry mature seeds of *Ligustrum lucidum* Ait., containing oleanolic acid and Usolic acid; and Rhizoma Cibotii is the dry rhizome of *Cibotium barometz* (L.) J. Sm.

Description Capsules containing brown or deep – brown power. Taste, slightly sour.

Action To reinforce kidney and strengthen body.

Indications Lumbar soreness, foot lassitude, dizziness, tinnitus, cardiopalmus, impotence and spermatorrhea.

Usage and dosage 3 capsules, 3 times a day, 7 days for treatment, or taken when necessary.

Precaution Use with caution in pregnancy.

Specification 0.3g per capsule.

Storage Preserve in well – closed containers.

Experiment materials

Instrument: flasks (1000ml, 500ml), electric heating plate, vacuum filter, water baths, stainless – steel dishes, vacuum loft drier, mortar, sieves, capsule filler, balance, and disintegration testing apparatus.

Drug and reagents: Herba Epimedii, Fructus Rosae Laevigatae, Semen Cuscutae, Fructus Ligustri Lucidi (processed), and Rhizoma Cibotii (processed)

Experimental Method

1. Formulation

Herba Epimedii	225g
Fructus Rosae Laevigatae	135g
Semen Cuscutae	135g
Fructus Ligustri Lucidi (Processed)	135g
Rhizoma Cibotii (processed)	135g

(The quantity may be reduced for the student's exercise.)

2. Procedure

(1) Decoction Decoct the medicinal slices of Herba Epimedii, Fructus Rosae Laevigatae, and Semen Cuscutae with and appropriate quantity of water twice, 2 hours for the first time and 1.5 hours for the second time. Combine the decoctions, filter, and let stand for 8 ~ 12 hours.

(2) Pulverization Pulverize Fructus Ligustri Lucidi (processed) and Rhizoma Cibotii (processed), and pass through sieve No.6.

(3) Concentration Concentrate the filtrate to a liquid extract with a relative density of 1.16 ~ 1.18 (70 ~ 80℃).

(4) Granulating Add the powder to the liquid extract, mix well, and dry them below 80℃. Grind the dried mixture into granules through sieve No.5.

(5) Packing Pack them to make capsules.

3. Tests

Comply with the relative requirements.

4. Calculation

Calculate the extractive rate of the of Herba Epimedii, Fructus Rosae Laevigatae, and Semen Cuscutae; the content of each capsule; and the yield of capsules.

Questions

1. What advantages do capsules have, compared with other solid dosage forms?
2. Summarize the methods of capsular preparation and key operations in brief.

Reference

1. Pharmacopoeia Commission of PRC. Pharmacopoeia of People Republic of China. Volume I. Beijing: Chemical Industry Press. 2000, Appendix 11

2. The Stationary Office. British Pharmacopoeia (Volume II, 2000 Edition). London, 2002, 1655

3. Pharmacopoeia Commission of PRC. Pharmacopoeia of People Republic of China. Volume I. Beijing: Chemical Industry Press. 2000, 533

4. Pharmacopoeia Commission of PRC. Pharmacopoeia of People Republic of China (Supplement, 2000 Edition). Beijing: Chemical Industry Press. 2002, 17

5. Health Ministry of P.R.China. Drug Standard of TCM Formulations. Vol.4, 87

6. Health Ministry of P.R.China. Drug Standard of Tibet. Vol.1, 73

实验十一　散　　剂

【实验目的】

通过六一散的制备，掌握中药散剂的制备方法、制剂特点及要求。

【实验指导】

散剂[1]系指一种或多种药材混合制成的粉末状制剂，可分为内服散剂和外用散剂。散剂历代应用颇多，迄今仍然为常用剂型之一。

1．制备散剂的一般要求

散剂在生产与贮藏期间均应符合下列有关规定：

（1）供制散剂的药材均应粉碎。一般散剂应为细粉，儿科及外用散剂应为最细粉号筛。

（2）散剂应干燥、疏松、混合均匀、色泽一致。如含有毒、剧毒药或贵重药的散剂时，应采用等量递增配研法混匀并过筛。

（3）用于烧伤或严重损伤的外用散剂，应在清洁避菌环境下配制并进行灭菌处理。

（4）一般散剂应密闭贮藏，含挥发性药物或易吸潮药物的散剂应密封贮藏。

2．散剂的检查

（1）均匀度检查

取供试品适量置光滑纸上，平铺约 5cm^2，将其表面压平，在亮处观察，应呈现均匀的色泽，无花纹、色斑。

（2）水分检查

烘干法：取供试品 2～5g，平铺于干燥至恒重的扁形称瓶中，厚度不超过 5mm，疏松样品不超过 10mm，精密称定，打开瓶盖在 100～105℃干燥 5 小时，将瓶盖盖好，移置干燥器中，冷却 30 分钟，精密称定重量，再在上述温度干燥 1 小时，冷却，称重，至连续两次称重的差异不超过 5mg 为止。根据减失的重量，计算供试品中含有水分的百分数，不得超过 9.0%。

（3）装量和装量检查

单剂量、一日剂量包装的散剂装量差异限度应符合下表规定：

标示装量	装量差异限度
0.1g 或 0.1g 以下	±15%
0.1g 以上至 0.5g	±10%
0.5g 以上至 1.5g	±8%
1.5g 以上至 6g	±7%
6g 以上	±5%

检查法：取供试品 10 袋（瓶），分别称定每袋（瓶）内容物的重量，每袋（瓶）的重

量与标示装量相比较，超出限度的不得多于2袋（瓶），并不得有1袋（瓶）超出限度一倍。未规定用量的外用散剂和非单剂量的大规格包装散剂不检查装量差异。

实验 六 一 散

六一散（Liuyi san）来源于古方，是治疗暑湿之常用方。本品收载于《中国药典》[2]。方中重用滑石甘淡性寒，清热利尿，使湿热从小便而出为君药，又佐甘草泻火和中，又可缓和滑石之寒太过，因滑石与甘草的比例为6∶1，且作散剂使用，故名“六一散”。

性状：本品为浅黄白色的粉末；具甘草甜味，手捻有润滑感。

功能与主治：清暑利湿。内服用于暑热身倦，口渴泄泻，小便黄少；外治痱子刺痒。

用法与用量：调服或包煎服，一次6~9g，一日1~2次；外用，扑撒患处。

贮藏：密闭，防潮。

【实验材料】

仪器：普通天平、研钵、筛子（五号、六号）、称量纸。

药品和试剂：甘草、滑石粉。

【实验方法】

1．处方

滑石粉	600g
甘草	100g

2．制法

(1) 称取甘草适量（大于60g），置于研钵中研磨成细粉，过筛。

(2) 称取过滤后的甘草细粉60g，置于研钵中，加入滑石粉适量，混匀，过筛，分装成袋，即得。

3．检查

应符合散剂的有关要求。

【思考题】

1．该散剂的有效成分是什么？

2．如何保证散剂的卫生学要求？

参 考 文 献

1．国家药典委员会．中华人民共和国药典（一部）．北京：化学工业出版社．2000，附录6

2．国家药典委员会．中华人民共和国药典（一部）．北京：化学工业出版社．2000，412

Exercise 11 Powder

Exercise objectives

1. Learn the general process to produce powders made from TCM drugs.
2. Understand the characteristics and requirements of powders.

Instruction

Powders[1] may be defined as mixtures as one or more kinds of pulverized crude drugs which are used for oral administration or externally application. Powders have been used for thousands of years. They are still one of dosage forms in common use.

1. General requirements for powder – preparation

The production and storage of powders should comply with the following requirements:

(1) The crude drugs for powders production should be comminuted. In general, powders should be fine powders, and powders for paediatrics and topical application should be very fine powders.

(2) Powders should be dry, loose, well mixed and uniform in appearance and colour. If they contain poisonous, potent, or precious drugs, they should be prepared by compounding and grinding methods with isochoric increase by degrees, mixed well and sifted.

(3) Powders for topical application of burns and severe wounds should be made under clean, sterile conditions and sterilized.

(4) Powders should be stored in well – closed containers. Powders containing volatile or moisture – absorbing drugs should be stored in tightly closed containers.

2. Tests

(1) The examination of uniformity

Spread evenly a sufficient quantity of powders in an area of about 5cm^2 on a piece of smooth paper, press the surface to be even, observe the powder under a bright light. It should be uniform in colouration without discolourations and stains.

(2) Determination of Water

Drying in oven method: Place 2 ~ 5 g of the substances being examined in a flat weighing bottle, previously dried to constant weight, to form a smooth layer not exceeding 5 mm in thickness, or not exceeding 10 mm in thickness for substance of loose texture. Dry at 100 ~ 105℃ for 5 hours, cover the weighing bottle, place it in a desiccator and allow it to cool for 30 minutes. Weigh accurately, dry it again under similar condition or 1 hour, cool and weigh. Repeat the operation until the difference between two successive weighings is not more than 5 mg. Calculate the percentage content of water in the substance being examined according to the weight loss on drying. The powders contain not more than 9.0% of water.

(3) Packing variation

Packing variation limit for powders presented in single or daily doses should comply with the requirements stated in the table below:

Labelled weight per pack (or vial)	Weight variation limit
0.1g or less than 0.1g	±15%
More than 0.1g to 0.5g	±10%
More than 0.5g to 1.5g	±8%
More than 1.5g to 6g	±7%
More than 6g	±5%

Procedure: Weigh accurately each of ten packs (or vials) of powders and compare the weight of the content of each with the labelled weight. Not more than 2 packs should exceed the packing variation limit and none should double the packing variation limit. It is unnecessary to examine the weight variation for powders applied externally of unspecified dose or large package powders of multiple doses.

Liuyi Powders

Liu yi powder comes from traditional formulations, collected in Pharmacopoeia of the People's Republic of China[2]. It is a common formula for syndrome of summer – heat and dampness. Being sweet flavor and cold nature, Pulvis Talci as the main ingredient clears heat and induces diuresis to disperse damp – heat out through urine. As the assistant herb, Radix Glycyrrhizae can purge fire and harmonize the middle as well as mitigate the coldness of Pulvis Talci. Since the proportion of Pulvis Talci and Radix Glycyrrhizae was 6:1, and the dosage form was powder, liu yi powders was named.

Description: A pale yellow – white powder; taste, characteristic sweet of Radix Glycyrrhizae, unctuous to touch.

Action and Indications: To remove summer – damp, lassitude, thirst, diarrhea and oliguria with deep – coloured urine after exposure to summer – heat; also used as heat – rash powder externally.

Usage and Dosage: 6 ~ 9g, 1 ~ 2 times a day, to be taken after mixing with liquids or making decoction with the drug wrapped with a piece of cloth or gauze; appropriate quantity to be dabbed on the affected part externally.

Storage: Preserve in well closed containers, protected from moisture.

Exercise Materials

Instruments: balance, mortar, sieve (NO.6), some pieces of weighing paper.

Drugs and reagents: Pulvis Talci, Radix Glycyrrhizae.

Exercise Methods

1. Formulation

Pulvis Talci	600g
Radix Glycyrrhizae	100g

2. Procedures

(1) Weigh Radix Glycyrrhizae (more than 60g), put them into mortar. Then grind them into fine powder, pass through sieves.

(2) Weigh accurately Radix Glycyrrhizae that have been sifted (60g), put into mortar, then add into Pulvis Talci (10g), mix them well, sift with sieves, and pack into bags.

3. Tests

Comply with the relative requirements.

Questions

1. What are the active ingredients in the powders?

2. How can we meet the requirements of sanitization for powder – preparation?

Reference

1. Pharmacopoeia commission of PRC. Pharmacopoeia of the People's Republic of China Volume I. Beijing: Chemistry Industry Press. 2000, Appendix 6.

2. Pharmacopoeia commission of PRC. Pharmacopoeia of the People's Republic of China Volume I. Beijing: Chemistry Industry Press. 2000, 412.

实验十二　灸　　剂

【实验目的】

通过药艾条的制备，掌握中草药灸剂的一般制法。

【实验指导】

灸剂是将艾叶捣碎如绒状，添加或不添加其他药料，制成一定大小形状后，可点燃熏灼，发散药味，置于体表的某些腧穴或患部，使之发生温热或灼痛感觉，并可吸收发散的药物成分，以达到预防或治疗目的的一种外用制剂。

艾绒的制法：取干燥的艾叶，拣去杂质，筛去尘土，置粉碎机或石臼、碾床中粉碎成棉绒状，除去叶脉，即得。

实验　药　艾　条

药艾条（Yao'aitiao）是中华人民共和国药典收载的一种灸剂[1]。药艾条的主要成分是艾叶。艾叶为艾蒿 Artemisiae Argyi 的干燥叶，含大量挥发油。

性状：本品呈圆柱状，长 20～21cm，直径 1.7～1.8cm；气香，点燃后发出持久的、气特异的烟，而不熄灭。

功能与主治：行气血，逐寒湿。用于风寒湿痹，肌肉酸麻，关节四肢疼痛，脘腹冷痛。

用法与用量：直射灸法，一次适量，红晕为度，一日 1～2 次；或遵医嘱。

规格：每支约重 30g。

贮藏：密闭，防潮。

【实验材料】

仪器：粉碎机。

药品和试剂：艾叶、桂枝、高良姜、广藿香、降香、香附、白芷、陈皮、丹参、生川乌，白棉纸（28×15cm），胶水。

【实验方法】

1．处方

艾叶	2400g	桂枝	125g	高良姜	125g
广藿香	50g	降香	175g	香附	50g
白芷	100g	陈皮	50g	丹参	50g
生川乌	75g				

（学生实验采用五十分之一量）

2．制法

以上十味，艾叶碾成艾绒，其余桂枝等八味粉碎成细粉，过筛，混匀。先取艾绒20g，均匀平铺在一张长28cm，宽15cm的白棉纸上，再均匀散布上述粉末8g，将棉纸两端折叠约6cm，卷紧成条，粘合封闭，低温干燥，即得。

3．检查

检查药艾条样品的性状，应符合规定的要求。

【思考题】

1．在制备过程中，为什么要采取低温干燥？

参考文献

1．中华人民共和国药典委员会．《中华人民共和国药典（一部）》（2000版）北京：化学工业出版社．516

Exercise 12 Moxa – preparation

Learning objectives

Learn and practice the common manufacturing procedure through preparation of yaoaitiao moxa rolls.

Instruction

Moxa – preparation is a dosage form for external application made by pulverizing Chinese mugwort leaves into mugwort floss, with or without other crude drug powders, and making into different shapes. In practice a lighted moxa is applied over the selected points of the affected parts of the body from certain distance to cause a mild warmth or burning sensation, while the evaporated constituents in it can be absorbed. It is used either for preventive or therapeutic purpose.

Preparation of moxa floss: Clear the impurities from dry moxa leaves and sift the leaves from earth. Smash the moxa leaves with a pulverizer or a mortar or a roller mill, and get rid of veins in the floss.

Yao' aitiao moxa rolls

Yao' aitiao moxa roll[1] is a preparation of Chinese traditional medicine, recorded in the Pharmacopoeia of the People's Republic of China. Folium Artemisiae Argyi is a main ingredient, containing a great deal of essential oil.

Description Cylindrical, 20 ~ 21cm long, 1.7 ~ 1.8cm in diameter; odour, aromatic; smoked persistently with characteristic odour after burning.

Action To promote the flow of qi and blood, and expel cold – damp.

Indications Rheumatic arthralgia, aching of muscles accompanied by numbness, epigastric or abdominal pain with cold sensation.

Usage and dosage To be applied for direct moxibustion until the appearance of glow. 1 ~ 2 times a day or following a physician's advice.

Specification About 30 g per roll.

Storage Preserve in well closed containers, protected from moisture.

Exercise materials

Instruments: Pestle, mortar, grinding mill, microscope.

Drugs and reagents: Folium Artemisiae Argyi; Ramus Cinnamomi; Rhizoma Alpiniae Officinarum; Herbs Pogostemonis; Lignum Dalbergiae Odoriferae; Rhizoma Cyperi; Radix Angelicae Dahuricae ; Pericarpium Citri Reticulatae; Radix Salviae Miltiorrhizae; Radix Aconiti (not prepared), white cotton – paper (28 × 15cm), and gluewater.

Exercise method

1. Prescription

Folium Artemisiae Argyi	2400g
Ramus Cinnamomi	125g
Rhizoma Alpiniae Officinarum	125g
Herbs Pogostemonis	50g
Lignum Dalbergiae Odoriferae	175g
Rhizoma Cyperi	50g
Radix Angelicae Dahuricae	100g
Pericarpium Citri Reticulatae	50g
Radix Salviae Miltiorrhizae	50g
Radix Aconiti (not prepared)	75g

Fiftieth for the student's exercise.

2. Procedure

Triturate *Folium Artemisiae Argyri* to tiny pieces. Pulverize all the other ingredients to fine powders, sift and mix well. Spread homogeneously 20 g of the tiny pieces of *Folium Artemisiae Argyri* on a sheet of white cotton – paper of 28cm in length and 15cm in width and scatter evenly 8g of the above power on it. Fold the cotton paper from two sides for 6 cm, roll with the paper to make sticks of drugs, seal, and dry at a lower temperature.

3. Test

The description of the sample should comply with the requirements of yaoaitiao moxa rolls.

Question

1. Why should the products of yaoaitiao moxa rolls be dried at a lower temperature?

Reference

1. Pharmacopoeia Commission of PRC. Pharmacopoeia of the People's Republic of China (English Edition), Volume Ⅰ, Beijing: Chemical Industry Press, 1997: 421 ~ 422

实验十三　滴　　丸

【实验目的】

1．熟悉中药滴丸剂的一般制法。

2．了解滴丸剂的特点。

【实验指导】

滴丸剂[1]系指固体或液体药物与基质加热熔化混匀后，滴入不相溶的冷凝液中，收缩冷凝而制成的制剂。药材须经过提取和精制后制成滴丸。

1．制备和贮藏中药滴丸一般要求

(1) 作为滴丸基质应具备下列条件：与主药不发生任何化学反应；对人体无害；熔点较低，加热易熔化成液体，而遇骤冷又能凝结成固体，在室温下保持固体状态。与主药混合后同样能保持以上物理状态。

基质包括水溶性基质和非水溶性基质，常用的水溶性基质有聚乙二醇 4000（或 6000)、硬脂酸钠、甘油明胶等。非水溶性基质有硬脂酸、单硬脂酸、蜂蜡、虫蜡、氢化油及植物油等。

(2) 冷凝液必须安全无害；不溶解主药和基质，不与之发生化学反应；密度与液滴相近，使滴丸在冷却液中缓缓下沉或上浮，充分凝固。

常用的冷却液：水溶性基质可用液体石蜡、植物油、甲基硅油、煤油等。脂肪性基质可用水或者不同浓度乙醇等。

(3) 滴丸应表面光滑、大小均一、色泽一致。

(4) 根据药物的性质与使用、贮藏的要求，在滴制成丸后可包糖衣或薄膜衣。

(5) 滴丸剂一般宜密封贮存，防止受潮、发霉、变质。

2．滴丸的检查

(1) 重量差异

滴丸剂重量差异限度应符合下表规定：

滴丸剂重量差异限度

每份标示量或平均重量	重量差异限度
0.1g 以下至 0.1g	±11%
0.1g 以上至 0.3g	±10%
0.3g 以上至 1g	±8%
1g 以上	±7%

检查法：以供试品 10 丸为 1 份，取 10 份，分别称定重量，再与标示重量或平均重量比较，超出重量差异限度不得多于 2 份，并不得有 1 份超出限度一倍。包衣滴丸应在包衣前检查丸芯的重量差异，符合上表规定后，方可以包衣。包衣后不再检查重量差异。

（2）溶散时限

《中华人民共和国药典》规定了一种滴丸剂溶散时限的检查法。

检查装置：采用升降式崩解仪，主要结构为一能升降的金属支架与下端镶有筛网的吊篮，并附有挡板。①支架：升降的金属支架上下移动距离为55mm±2mm，往返频率为每分钟30~32次。②吊篮：玻璃管6根，管长77.5mm±2.5mm，内径21.5mm，壁厚2mm，透明塑料板2块，直径90mm，厚6mm，板面有6个孔，孔径26mm；不锈钢板1块（放在上面一块塑料板上），直径90mm，厚1mm，板面有6个孔，孔径22mm；不锈钢丝筛网1张（放在下面一块塑料板下），直径90mm，筛孔内径0.425mm；以及不锈钢轴1根（固定在上面一块塑料板与不锈钢板上），长80mm；将上述玻璃管6根垂直于2块塑料板的孔中，并用3只螺丝将不锈钢板、塑料板和不锈钢丝筛网固定，即得。③挡板：为一平整光滑得透明塑料块，相对密度1.18~1.20，直径20.7mm±0.15mm，厚9.5mm±0.15mm；挡板共有5个孔，孔径2mm，中央1个孔，其余4个孔距中心6mm，各孔间距相等；挡板侧边有4个等距离的V型槽，V型槽上端宽9.5mm，深2.55mm，底部开口处的宽与深度均为1.6mm。

检查方法：将吊篮通过上端的不锈钢轴悬挂于金属支架上，浸入1000ml烧杯中，并调节吊篮位置使其下降时筛网间距烧杯底部25mm，烧杯中盛有温度为37℃±1℃的水，调节水位高度使吊篮上升时筛网在水面下25mm处。除另有规定外，取供试品6粒，分别置于上述吊篮的玻璃管中，加挡板，启动崩解仪进行检查，应在30分钟内全部溶散，包衣滴丸应在1小时内全部溶散。如有1粒不能完全溶散，应另取6粒复试。均应符合规定。以明胶为基质的滴丸，可改在人工胃液中进行检查。

实验　穿心莲内酯滴丸的制备

穿心莲和穿心莲片是《中华人民共和国药典》收载的中药，具有清热解毒，凉血消肿的功效。穿心莲内酯（andrographolide）是其主要有效成分，为难溶性二萜化合物。将穿心莲内酯制成滴丸有利于其溶出。根据中国专利报道，已经有成熟的穿心莲内酯滴丸的工艺。本实验课依据该专利说明书的配方和基本工艺进行实验练习。

【实验材料】

仪器：滴丸装置、普通电炉、烧杯（500ml、1000ml）、玻璃棒、量筒、漏斗、温度计、滤纸、分析天平、崩解仪等。

药品和试剂材料：穿心莲内酯、穿心莲内酯片、聚乙二醇6000、硬脂酸、二甲基硅油等。

【实验方法】

1．配方

穿心莲内酯	50g
聚乙二醇6000	350g
硬脂酸	15g

（学生实验可用十分之一量）

2．制法

（1）药液的配制　取 PEG_{6000} 35g 和硬脂酸 1.5g，加热熔融，加入穿心莲内酯 5g，搅拌均匀。

（2）滴制　①趁热将药液倒入滴丸滴制装置（见示意图）的药液管中，调节水浴温度，使药液温度恒定于 80℃。②将二甲基硅油装入置于冰浴环境中的冷凝瓶中。③调节活塞，使药液以适当的速度滴入冷却液中；可适当轻轻晃动冷却液，以免成型滴丸局部堆积。

（3）收集　滴制完成后，回收冷却液，取出滴丸，用滤纸吸干滴丸表面的冷却液，晾干。

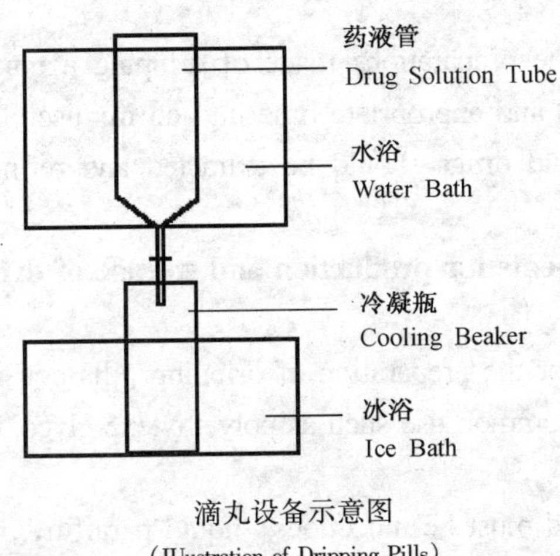

滴丸设备示意图

（IUustration of Dripping Pills）

3．检查

(1) 依法进行重量差异和溶散时限检查。

(2) 依照崩解时限检查法检查穿心莲内酯片的崩解时限。

【思考题】

1．比较片剂和滴丸的特点。

2．为何滴丸剂疗效迅速、生物利用度高？

参　考　文　献

1．国家药典委员会．中华人民共和国药典（一部）．北京：化学工业出版社．2000，附录11

2．许军，钱进，刘智等．穿心莲内酯滴丸及其制备方法．中国专利申请号 03110092.9．2003 年 10 月1 日

Exercise 13 Dripping Pills

Learning objectives

1. Known the specific properties of dripping pills.

2. Learn and practice the common process of preparation dripping pills of traditional Chinese medicine.

Instruction

Dripping pills[1] are the preparations made of dripping a uniform, melted mixture of solid or liquid medicaments and appropriate base into an immiscible cooling liquid and congealing to a pill form. Crud drugs should be extracted and refined for preparation of the pills.

1. General requirements for production and storage of dripping pills of traditional Chinese medicine.

(1) The bases used for the preparation of dripping pills consist of water – soluble and water – insoluble bases in common use such as polyethylene glycol 6000, gelatin and stearic acid.

(2) The cooling liquid must be innocuous; liquid paraffin, vegetable oil, methylsilicone oil and water are commonly used for this purpose.

(3) Dripping pills should be uniform in size and colour.

(4) Dripping pills may be sugar – coated or film – coated as required to suit for the properties of the medicaments and for the clinical usage and storage.

(5) Unless otherwise specified dripping pills should be kept in tightly closed containers, protected from moisture, mold and prevented from deterioration.

2. Tests

(1) Weight variation The limit of weight variation for dripping pills complied with the following requirements.

Labelled weight or average weight	Limit of weight variation
Less than 0.1g and 0.1g	±11%
More than 0.1g and 0.3g	±10%
More than 0.3g and 1g	±8%
More than 1g	±7%

Procedure Take 10 portions of pills. Weigh the weight of each portion containing 10 pills. Compare the weight with the labelled weight or average of portions. Not more than 2 portions deviate outside the limit of weight variation, none deviates outside 1 fold of the limit. The weight variation of coated dripping pills should be examined before coating. Dripping pills are not to be coated until the weight variation of their cores complies with the requirements stated in the table above.

(2) Disintegration test Appendix of Pharmacopoeia of the People's Republic of China specified a method for determination of disintegration.

Apparatus: The apparatus mainly consists of a basket – rack assembly with disk and a motion device for raising and lowing.

①motion device: The motion device for raising and lowing the basket in the liquid medium at a constant rate between 30 ~ 32 cycles per minute through a distance of 55mm ± 2mm. ②Basket rack assembly: The basket – rack assembly consists of six glass tube, each 77.5mm ± 2.5mm long, 21.5mm in the internal diameter with a wall of 2mm thickness. The tubes are held in a vertical position by two transparent plastic plates, each about 90mm in diameter and 6mm in thickness, with six holes, each about 26mm in diameter. On the top of the upper layer plate is a stainless steel plate about 90mm in diameter and 1mm in thickness, with six holes each about 22mm in diameter. Attached to the under surface of the lower plate is a disk of stainless – steel wire gauze about 90mm in diameter, with apertures of 0.425mm in internal fixed with the upper plastic plate and stainless – steel plate. The stainless – steel plate, the two plastic plates and the wire gauze are fixed together by three screws. ③ disks: The disks are about 9.5mm ± 0.15mm thick and 20.7mm ± 0.15mm in diameter, made of a smooth, transparent plastic material having a specific gravity of 1.18 ~ 1.20. It has five holes with 2mm in diameter, one of the holes is located in the center and the others at an equal distance of 6mm from the central hole. Equally spaced on the sides of the disk are four V – shaped notches. The dimensions of each notch are such that the upper openings are 9.5mm wide and 2.55mm deep and lower openings are 1.6mm wide and 1.6mm deep.

Procedure: The basket is suspended in a 1000ml beaker, maintained at 37℃ ± 1℃, the volume of the fluid in the vessel is adjusted appropriately so that at the highest point of the upward stroke the wire mesh remains at least 25mm below the surface of the fluid and descends to a distance not less than 25mm from the bottom of the vessel on downward stroke. Unless otherwise specified, place 1pill in each of the 6 tubes of the basket, add a disk and operate the apparatus. Pills disintegrate completely within 30 minutes; coated pills disintegrate completely within 1hour. If 1 pill fails to disintegrate completely, repeat the operation with another 6 pills. All the pills should comply with the test. Dripping pills made of gelatin base may be tested in simulated gastric fluid.

Preparation of Andrographolide Dripping Pills

Herba Andrographis and Tabellae Andrographis are drugs of Chinese traditional medicine recorded in the Pharmacopoeia of The People's Republic of China (Volume Ⅰ), which can remove heat, counteract toxicity, and induce subsidence of swelling. Andrographolide is an active ingredient in these drugs, but slightly soluble. A preparation of dripping pills is invented, reported by Chinese Patent[2], which may help increase the solubility rate of andrographolide. According to the formulation and its basic procedure described in the report, we exercise to make andrographolide dripping pills.

Exercise materials

Instruments: Apparatus of dropping pills, beaker (500ml, 100ml), glasses stick, measuring cylinder, funnel, thermometer, filter paper, analytical balance, and disintegration apparatus.

Drug and Reagents Material andrographolide, andrographolide tablets, PEG6000, stearic acid, and dimethyl silicone oil.

Exercise methods

1. Formulation

andrographolide	50g
PEG6000	350g
stearic acid	15g

(A tenth for the student's exercise.)

2. Procedure

(1) Preparation of drug solution Melt PEG_{6000} 35g and stearic acid 1.5g together, add 5g of andrographolide to dissolve, keeping hot.

(2) Dripping ①Add the drug solution into the drug solution tube, and adjust the temperature of water bath to 80℃. ② Add dimethyl silicone oil into cooling beaker in an ice bath. ③Adjust the valve carefully to a satisfactory dripping speed. Shake the cool liquid gently to prevent the dripping pills from agglomerating.

(3) Collection Filter, blot up the remainder of the cool liquid with filter paper. Dry the pills in air.

3. Tests

(1) Carry out the disintegration test and the weight variation test as described above.

(2) Carry out the test to determinate disintegration of andrographolide tablets.

Question

1. Compare properties of tablets with dripping pills.

2. Why do the dripping pills cause curative effect more quickly and enhance its bioavailability?

Reference

1. Pharmacopoeia Commission of PRC. Pharmacopoeia of the People's Republic of China (English Edition), Volume Ⅰ. Beijing: Chemical Industry Press. 1997, Appendix A-8

2. Xu Jun, Qian Jin, Liu Zhi, etc. Andrographolide dripping pills and its manufacture method. Chinese Patent Application Number 03110092.9. Oct. 1, 2003.

实验十四　环糊精包合物和制剂设计

【实验目的】

1. 学习环糊精包合物制备方法。
2. 学习设计一种草药制剂。

【实验指导】

薄荷（*Metha haplocalyx* Brig）是一种广泛用于医药和烹调的草药。薄荷油是一种从新鲜的薄荷茎叶中用水蒸汽蒸馏出来挥发油后，再经过冷冻和除去部分薄荷脑（menthol）之后所得到的油。薄荷叶含有大约0.1%～1.0%的挥发油，其最主要的组分是薄荷脑（以及薄荷酮（menthone））。

中国药典规定薄荷油（Oleum menthae）应符合下列标准[1]：含酯量，按醋酸薄荷酯计算，不得少于2.0%（w/w）和不得大于6.5%（w/w）；总醇量，按薄荷脑计算，不得少于50%（w/w）。

薄荷油是一种祛风药、芳香剂和调味料。用于皮肤黏膜能产生清凉的感觉，可以减轻不适和疼痛。薄荷油通常在西方国家用于治疗各种消化不适，可以缓解消化道痉挛。

薄荷油（Oleum menthae）用法和剂量：口服，一次0.02～0.2 ml；一日0.06～0.6 ml。外用适量。

薄荷油可以制成各种剂型，例如肠衣制剂、口含片、芳香水剂、软膏和微囊。含有挥发性物质的固体应该有适当地保护措施以免由于受热和长期储存遭受损失。环糊精包合物技术可以用于固化挥发性物质。

环糊精（cyclodextrin，简称CD）是一种由吡喃葡萄糖单位连接的环状寡聚糖。α，β，γ环糊精分别由6、7、8个吡喃葡萄糖组成，其中两个吡喃葡萄糖之间由α－（1，4）糖苷键连接形成筒状。环糊精可与固体、液体或气体分子形成固态的结晶的复合物。具有合适的大小和形状的分子进入环糊精的孔穴中形成包合物。环糊精是一种“分子囊”，具有疏水的内部和亲水的外部。β环糊精由于其分子的空间结构和便宜的价格在药学有重要的实际意义。在包合物中的难溶性疏水分子的溶解度可以提高。因此，其溶出速度也能提高。环糊精包合能将一种液体物质转变成一种固体复合物并且固定芳香物质和挥发性药物。

实验　薄荷油β－环糊精包合物

练习用薄荷油制备β－CD包合物。

【实验材料】

仪器：具塞锥型瓶（100ml）、磁力搅拌器、布氏漏斗、干燥器、挥发油提取器、TLC

仪器。

药品和试剂：β－环糊精、无水乙醇、薄荷油、乙酸乙酯、石油醚、香草醛、硫酸。

【实验方法】

1．处方

β－CD	4g
薄荷油	1ml（28d）
水	50ml

2．制法

称取β－CD4g，放入100ml的带塞瓶中，加入50ml水，加热溶解，降温至50℃，加入薄荷油1ml，加热搅拌2.5小时，保持50℃，过滤，用无水乙醇5ml洗涤三次，至表面近无油香，将包合物置于干燥器中。

3．检查

（1）差示热分析。

（2）测定包合率　取包合物3g，置250ml圆底烧瓶中加水150ml，用挥发油提取器提取挥发油，测β－CD的包合率（参见《中国药典》附录之挥发油测定法）。按下表计算包合率。

W_1产品总量	g
W_2测试的产品量	g
W_3用去的挥发油总量	g
W_4从测试的产品提取的挥发油量	g

$$包合率（\%）=\frac{W_4 \times W_1}{W_3 \times W_2} \times 100$$

（3）鉴别

① 样品的制备：A．取包合物0.5g，加入95%乙醇2ml，溶解、过滤的溶液作为测试品溶液。B．取薄荷油2滴，加入95%乙醇2ml，溶解所得的溶液作为对照品溶液。

② 薄层层析：照《中国药典》规定的薄层层析法，采用含有羧甲基纤维素钠的硅胶G薄层板，吸取分别2μl两种溶液点于薄层板上，以乙酸乙酯－石油醚（15:85，V/V）为展开剂展开。展开结束后，移出薄层板，在空气中晾干，喷1%香草醛硫酸溶液，加热显色。

实验　薄荷油制剂设计

试设计一种薄荷油制剂，包括以下内容：

1．前言，介绍有关薄荷油的背景和你的新思路。

2．制剂处方，包括你拟设计的制剂的所有成分的名称和数量以及用这些材料制备的成品的数量。

3．实验方法，包括制备成品的每一步操作。

4．材料，包括你的试验所需要的仪器、药品和试剂。

5．检查，控制成品质量的测定方法。

6．标签，应符合国家食品药品管理局规定的有关要求。

7．参考文献，记录你为了该设计所阅读和应用的已发表的文献。

【思考题】

1．形成包合物的关键是什么?

2．使用环糊精包合物在药剂学上有何意义?

参 考 文 献

1. 国家药典委员会．中华人民共和国药典（一部）．北京：化学工业出版社．2000，310

Exercise 14 Cyclodextrin Inclusion Complexes and Preparation Design

Learning objectives

1. Learn preparation of cyclodextrin inclusion complexes.
2. Design an herb formulation proposal.

Introduction

Peppermint (*Metha haplocalyx* Brig.) is a widely used herb for both medicinal and culinary purposes. Peppermint oil is the volatile oil by steam distillation from the fresh stem and leaf of peppermint. The oil obtained is cooled, removed partly from menthol. Peppermint leaves yield approximately 0.1% ~ 1.0% volatile oil which is composed primarily of menthol and menthone.

The Chinese Pharmacopoeia specifies that peppermint oil (Oleum menthae) should be standardized to that it is not less than 2.0% (w/w) and not more than 6.5% (w/w) of esters calculated as menthyl acetate; not less than 50% (w/w) of free alcohols calculated as menthol.

Peppermint oil is classified as a carminative, and aromatic, flavouring agent. Apply to the skin or mucous membrane to give cooling feeling, and to relieve pain or other uncomfortable symptom. The oil of peppermint is used routinely in western countries to treat a variety of digestive complaints. It may relieve spasms in the intestinal tract.

Usage and Dosage of Oleum menthae 0.02 ~ 0.2 ml; 0.06 ~ 0.6 ml daily.

Peppermint oil may be prepared in various dosage forms, such as enteric coated preparation, buccal and sublingual tablets, aromatic waters, ointments, and microcapsules. Solid preparations containing volatile substances should be protected from loss due to heating or long – term storage. Technology of cyclodextrin inclusion has been used for fixation of volatile substances.

Cyclodextrins (CDs) are cyclic oligosaccharides built up from glucopyranose units. α, β, γCDs have 6, 7, 8 glucopyranose units respectively, in which α – (1, 4) glycosidic linkage of two glucopyranose units forms truncated cone shape. CDs form solid, crystalline complexes with solid, liquid or gaseous guest molecules. Molecules of appropriate size and shape fit into the CD cavity to form inclusion complexes. CDs are 'molecular capsules' with a hydrophobic inside and a hydrophilic outside. β – CD has practical importance in pharmacy because of its molecular dimensions and price. Solubility of sparingly soluble hydrophobic molecules can be enhanced in inclusion complexes. Hence the dissolution rate can also be increased. CD inclusion converts a liquid substrate to a solid complex and fix aroma – containing substances and volatile drugs.

Peppermint Oilβ – CD Inclusion Complex

Prepare of β – CD inclusion complex with peppermint oil.

Exercise materials

Instruments: Conical flask with stopper (100ml), porcelain funnel, magnetic stirrer, desiccator, steam distillation apparatus, and TLC apparatus.

Drugs and reagents: β – cyclodextrin, ethanol, peppermint oil, acetyl acetate, petroleum ether, vanillaldehyde, and sulphuric acid.

(1) Formulation

β – CD	4g
Peppermint oil	1ml (28drops)
Water	50ml

(2) Procedure

Add 4g of β – CD in 50ml of water in a conical flask (100ml) with stopper, heat to dissolve β – CD, allow to cool to the temperature of 50℃, add 1ml of peppermint oil, stir for 2.5 hour at 50℃, filter and wash the filtrate with 5ml of absolute ethanol for three times to the peppermint smell disappeared, dry and store the product in a desiccators.

(3) Tests

- Differential thermo – analysis for determination of the complex forming
- Determination of inclusion rate

Add 3g of the product in 250 ml of water in a flask (250 ml), extract the volatile oil with a set of steam distillation apparatus (See the Ch.P.Appendix). The inclusion rate is calculated as follows:

W_1 Weight of total products	g
W_2 Weight of tested products	g
W_3 Weight of volatile oil useded totally	g
W_4 Weight of volatile oil extracted from the tested products	g

$$\text{Inclusion rate (\%)} = \frac{W_4 \times W_1}{W_3 \times W_2} \times 100$$

- Identification

Preparation of Sample: (A) Grind well 0.5g, add 2ml of 95% ethanol, stir and filter to produce a solution as the test solution. (B) Dissolve two drops of peppermint oil CRS in

2ml of 95% ethanol as the reference solution.

TLC: Carry out the method for thin layer chromatograph specified in the Chinese Pharmacopoeia, using silica gel G as the coating substance and acetyl acetate – petroleum ether (15:75) as mobile phase. Apply separately to the plate 2 μl of each of the two solutions. After developing and removal of the plate, dry it in air, spray with a 1% solution of vanillaldehyde in sulphuric acid and heat until the spots are distinct.

Design of Peppermint Oil Dosage Form

Try to design of a peppermint oil dosage form, including follow contents:

1. Introduction, including the background of peppermint oil and your new idea.
2. Formulation, including names and quantities of all ingredients used in the proposal dosage form, and quantity of the finished product to be made with the listed materials.
3. Laboratory procedure, including each step to prepare the finished product.
4. Materials, including instruments, drugs, and reagents you needed for the Exercise.
5. Tests to control the quality of the finished product.
6. Label, complying with requirements specified by the SFDA of China.
7. References, including the public literatures you read and used in your design paper.

Questions

1. What is the key to form an inclusion complex?
2. What are the benefits to a preparation using a CD – inclusion method?

Reference

1. The Pharmacopoeia commission of China. Pharmacopoeia of the People's Republic of China. Volume Ⅰ. Beijing: Chemistry Industry Press. 2000, 310.

附录一 药品包装、标签和说明书管理规定（暂行）

《药品包装、标签和说明书管理规定》（暂行）于2000年3月17日经国家食品药品监督管理局局务会审议通过，现予发布，自2001年1月1日起执行。

药品包装、标签和说明书管理规定（暂行）

第一条　为加强药品监督管理，规范药品的包装、标签及说明书，以利于药品的运输、贮藏和使用，保证人民用药安全有效，特制定本规定。

第二条　药品包装、标签及说明书必须按照国家食品药品监督管理局规定的要求印制，其文字及图案不得加入任何未经审批同意的内容。

第三条　药品包装内不得夹带任何未经批准的介绍或宣传产品、企业的文字、音像及其他资料。

第四条　凡在中国境内销售、使用的药品，其包装、标签及说明书所用文字必须以中文为主并使用国家语言文字工作委员会公布的规范化汉字。

第五条　药品的通用名称必须用中文显著标示，如同时有商品名称，则通用名称与商品名称用字的比例不得小于1:2，通用名称与商品名称之间应有一定空隙，不得连用。

第六条　药品商品名称须经国家食品药品监督管理局批准后方可在药品包装、标签及说明书上标注。

第七条　提供药品信息的标志及文字说明，字迹应清晰易辨，标示清楚醒目，不得有印字脱落或粘贴不牢等现象，并不得用粘贴、剪切的方式进行修改或补充。

第八条　药品的包装分内包装与外包装。

（一）内包装系指直接与药品接触的包装（如安瓿、注射剂瓶、铝箔等）。内包装应能保证药品在生产、运输、贮藏及使用过程中的质量，并便于医疗使用。

药品内包装材料、容器（药包材）的更改，应根据所选用药包材的材质，做稳定性试验，考察药包材与药品的相容性。

（二）外包装系指内包装以外的包装，按由里向外分为中包装和大包装。外包装应根据药品的特性选用不易破损的包装，以保证药品在运输、贮藏、使用过程中的质量。

第九条　药品的标签分为内包装标签与外包装标签。

（一）内包装标签与外包装标签内容不得超出国家食品药品监督管理局批准的药品说明书所限定的内容；文字表达应与说明书保持一致。

（二）内包装标签可根据其尺寸的大小，尽可能包含药品名称、适应证或者功能主治、用法用量、规格、贮藏、生产日期、生产批号、有效期、生产企业等标示内容，但必须标注药品名称、规格及生产批号。

（三）中包装标签应注明药品名称、主要成分、性状、适应证或者功能主治、用法用量、不良反应、禁忌证、规格、贮藏、生产日期、生产批号、有效期、批准文号、生产企业等内容。

（四）大包装标签应注明药品名称、规格、贮藏、生产日期、生产批号、有效期、批准文号、生产企业以及使用说明书规定以外的必要内容，包括包装数量、运输注意事项或其他标记等。

（五）标签上有效期具体表述形式应为：有效期至×年×月。

（六）由于尺寸原因，中包装标签不能全部注明不良反应、禁忌证、注意事项的，均应注明“详见说明书”字样。

第十条　原料药的包装参照本规定第八条第（一）项执行，标签按制剂大包装标签规定办理。

第十一条　药品的每个最小销售单元的包装必须按照规定印有或贴有标签并附有说明书。

第十二条　药品说明书应包含有关药品的安全性、有效性等基本科学信息。

药品的说明书应列有以下内容：药品名称（通用名、英文名、汉语拼音、化学名称、分子式、分子量、结构式（复方制剂、生物制品应注明成分）、性状、药理毒理、药代动力学、适应证、用法用量、不良反应、禁忌证、注意事项（孕妇及哺乳期妇女用药、儿童用药、药物相互作用和其他类型的相互作用，如烟、酒等）、药物过量（包括症状、急救措施、解毒药）、有效期、贮藏、批准文号、生产企业（包括地址及联系电话）等内容。如某一项目尚不明确，应注明“尚不明确”字样；如明确无影响，应注明“无”。

药品生产企业应主动跟踪药品上市后的应用情况，并在必要时提出修改说明书的申请。印制说明书，必须按照统一格式（说明书格式见附件一、二），其内容必须与国家食品药品监督管理局批准的说明书一致。

第十三条　药品的用法用量除单位含量标示外，还应使用通俗易懂的文字，如：“一次×片，一日×次”，“一次×支，一日×次”等，以正确指导用药。

第十四条　麻醉药品、精神药品、医疗用毒性药品、放射性药品等特殊管理的药品、外用药品、非处方药品在其中包装、大包装和标签、说明书上必须印有符合规定的标志；对贮藏有特殊要求的药品，必须在包装、标签的醒目位置和说明书中注明。

第十五条　药品的包装、标签及说明书在申请该药品注册时依药品的不同类别按照相应的管理规定办理审批手续。已注册上市的药品，凡修订或更改包装、标签或说明书的，均须按照原申报程序履行报批手续。

第十六条　凡违反本规定的，药品监督管理部门或者药品监督管理机构应责令药品生产企业更改其包装、标签或说明书、收回已上市的不符合本规定的药品。同时，按照《药品管理法》、《药品管理法实施办法》的有关规定予以处罚。

第十七条　本规定由国家食品药品监督管理局负责解释。

第十八条　本规定自 2001 年 1 月 1 日起执行。

附件一：

化学药品与生物制品说明书格式

××××说明书

【药品名称】
通用名：
商品名：
英文名：
汉语拼音：
本品主要成分及其化学名称为：
其结构式为：
分子式：
分子量：
（注：1．复方制剂应写为："本品为复方制剂，其组分为："
2．生物制品本项内容为主要组成成分。）
【性状】
【药理毒理】
【药代动力学】
【适应证】
【用法用量】
【不良反应】
【禁忌证】
【注意事项】
【孕妇及哺乳期妇女用药】
【儿童用药】
【老年患者用药】
【药物相互作用】
【药物过量】
【规格】
【有效期】
【贮藏】
【批准文号】
【生产企业】（地址、联系电话）

附件二：

中药说明书格式

××××说明书

【药品名称】
品　　名：
汉语拼音：
【性　　状】
【主要成分】
【药理作用】
【功能与主治】
【用法与用量】
【不良反应】
【禁忌证】
【注意事项】
【规　　格】
【贮　　藏】
【包　　装】
【有效期】
【批准文号】
【生产企业】（地址、联系电话）

附录二　药品包装、标签规范细则（暂行）

根据国家食品药品监督管理局第23号局令，进一步加强和规范药品的包装、标签管理，确保《药品包装、标签和说明书管理规定》（暂行）的贯彻实施，特制定本细则。

总体要求

一、药品包装、标签必须按照国家食品药品监督管理局规定的要求印制，其文字及图案不得加入任何未经审批同意的内容。药品的包装分为内包装和外包装。药品包装、标签内容不得超出国家食品药品监督管理局批准的药品说明书所限定的内容。

二、药品包装、标签上印刷的内容对产品的表述要准确无误，除表述安全、合理用药的用词外，不得印有各种不适当宣传产品的文字和标识，如“国家级新药”、“中药保护品种”、“GMP认证”、“进口原料分装”、“监制”、“荣誉出品”、“获奖产品”、“保险公司质量保险”、“公费报销”、“现代科技”、“名贵药材”等。

三、药品的商品名须国家食品药品监督管理局批准后方可在包装、标签上使用。商品名不得与通用名连写，应分行。商品名经商标注册后，仍须符合商品名管理的原则。通用名与商品名用字的比例不得小于1:2（指面积）。通用名字体大小应一致，不加括号。未经国家食品药品监督管理局批准作为商品名使用的注册商标，可印刷在包装标签的左上角或右上角，其字体不得大于通用名的用字。

四、同一企业，同一药品的相同规格品种（指药品规格和包装规格两种），其包装、标签的格式及颜色必须一致，不得使用不同的商标。同一企业的相同品种如有不同规格，其最小销售单元的包装、标签应明显区别或规格项应明显标注。

五、药品的最小销售单元，系指直接供上市药品的最小包装。每个最小销售单元的包装必须按照规定印有标签并附有说明书。

六、麻醉药品、精神药品、医疗用毒性药品、放射性药品等特殊管理的药品、外用药品、非处方药品在其大包装、中包装、最小销售单元和标签上必须印有符合规定的标志；对贮藏有特殊要求的药品，必须在包装、标签的醒目位置中注明。

七、进口药品的包装、标签除按本细则规定执行外，还应标明“进口药品注册证号”或“医药产品注册证号”、生产企业名称等；进口分包装药品的包装、标签应标明原生产国或地区企业名称、生产日期、批号、有效期及国内分包装企业名称等。

八、经批准异地生产的药品，其包装、标签还应标明集团名称、生产企业、生产地点；经批准委托加工的药品，其包装、标签还应标明委托双方企业名称、加工地点。

九、凡在中国境内销售和使用的药品，包装、标签所用文字必须以中文为主并使用国家语言文字工作委员会公布的现行规范文字。民族药可增加其民族文字。企业根据需要，在其药品包装上可使用条形码和外文对照；获我国专利的产品，亦可标注专利标记和专利号，并标明专利许可的种类。

十、包装标签有效期的表达方法，按年月顺序。一般表达可用有效期至某年某月，或只用数字表示。如有效期至2001年10月，或表达为有效期至2001．10、2001/10、2001－10等形式。年份要用四位数字表示，1至9月份数字前须加0以两位数表示月份。

各类药品包装、标签内容

一、化学药品与生物制品、制剂：

（一）内包装标签内容包括：

【药品名称】、【规格】、【适应证】、【用法用量】、【贮藏】【生产日期】、【生产批号】、【有效期】及【生产企业】。由于包装尺寸的原因而无法全部标明上述内容的，可适当减少，但至少须标注【药品名称】、【规格】、【生产批号】三项（如安瓿、滴眼剂瓶、注射剂瓶等）。

（二）直接接触内包装的外包装标签内容包括：

【药品名称】、【成分】、【规格】、【适应证】、【用法用量】、【贮藏】、【不良反应】、【禁忌证】、【注意事项】、【包装】、【生产日期】、【生产批号】、【有效期】、【批准文号】及【生产企业】。由于包装尺寸的原因而不能注明不良反应、禁忌证、注意事项，均应注明“详见说明书”字样。

对预防性生物制品，上述【适应证】项均应列为【接种对象】。

（三）大包装标签内容包括：

【药品名称】、【规格】、【生产批号】、【生产日期】、【有效期】、【贮藏】、【包装、【批准文号】、【生产企业】及运输注意事项或其他标记。

二、原料药标签内容包括：

【药品名称】、【包装规格】、【生产批号】、【生产日期】、【有效期】、【贮藏】、【批准文号】、【生产企业】及运输注意事项或其他标记。

三、中药制剂：

（一）内包装标签内容包括：

【药品名称】、【规格】、【功能与主治】、【用法用量】、【贮藏】、【生产日期】、【生产批号】、【有效期】及【生产企业】。因标签尺寸限制无法全部注明上述内容的，可适当减少，但至少须标注【药品名称】、【规格】、【生产批号】三项，如安瓿、注射剂瓶等。中药蜜丸蜡壳至少须标注【药品名称】。

（二）直接接触内包装的外包装标签内容包括：

【药品名称】、【成分】、【规格】、【功能与主治】、【用法用量】、【贮藏】、【不良反应】、【禁忌证】、【注意事项】、【包装】、【生产日期】、【生产批号】、【有效期】、【批准文号】及【生产企业】。由于包装尺寸的原因而不能注明不良反应、禁忌证、注意事项，均应注明“详见说明书”字样。

（三）大包装标签内容包括：

【药品名称】、【规格】、【生产批号】、【生产日期】、【有效期】、【贮藏】、【包装】、【批准文号】、【生产企业】及运输注意事项或其他标记。

本细则自颁布之日起施行。

本细则由国家食品药品监督管理局负责解释。

内 容 提 要

《中药制剂学实验与指导》汇编了各类中药制剂（固体、液体、半固体或分散体系）的普通代表性制剂或者制剂技术的实验内容。其中介绍的中药制剂基本上是具有国家标准的药物。选编这些实验供学生练习是为了说明和加强在课堂讲授的中药药剂学的基本概念，以便学生掌握各类制剂的化学、制备、质量控制和应用的基本要求。该书适用于本、专科试验教学，同时可供相关专业人员参考。

图书在版编目（CIP）数据

中药制剂学实验与指导/赵浩如主编．—北京：中国医药科技出版社，2004，9

普通高等教育“十一五”国家级规划教材　全国高等医药院校药学类实验教材

ISBN 978－7－5067－3047－1

Ⅰ．中…　Ⅱ．赵…　Ⅲ．中药制剂学－实验－医学院校－教学参考资料　Ⅳ．R283－33

中国版本图书馆 CIP 数据核字（2004）第 091580 号

美术编辑　陈君杞
责任校对　张学军
版式设计　郭小平

出版　中国医药科技出版社
地址　北京市海淀区文慧园北路甲 22 号
邮编　100082
电话　发行：010－62227427　邮购：010－62236938
网址　www. cmstp. com
规格　787×1092mm $^{1}/_{16}$
印张　9 $^{1}/_{4}$
字数　188 千字
版次　2004 年 10 月第 1 版
印次　2016 年 1 月第 3 次印刷
印刷　三河市双峰印刷装订有限公司
经销　全国各地新华书店
书号　ISBN 978－7－5067－3047－1
定价　15.00 元